What They're Saying About Empower Your Child To Heal

Dr. Hamilton provides a thorough and compelling book to help understand how anxiety cultivates disease. More importantly, she offers scientifically-proven ways to virtually eliminate conditions related to anxiety, gastrointestinal and autoimmune disorders. She proves the power of the mind is a wonder to behold.
— Dr. Mike Dow, Best-selling Author of *The Brain Fog Fix*, drmikedow.com

It's one of the most interesting books I have ever read, and I've been in publishing for more than 25 years, so that's really saying something. Her "Top 10 Things Kids Wish You Knew" hit me hard, and I mean that in a good way. I think every parent needs to read that list. The whole book was very eye opening. Dr. Skyler has a wonderful warm, friendly tone and comes across as very relatable. She distills complicated subject matter into prose that is easy to comprehend.
— Kathy Savadel, Book Editor

Dr. Skyler Hamilton opened my eyes to the correlation between anxiety and physical illness, and more importantly, how to heal from those conditions. Her well-researched argument, candid advice, personal and professional anecdotes offer the reader tangible and powerful strategies that will surely offer many parents hope and help. I'm sure I'll be passing along *Empower Your Child To Heal* to my clients as well. Well done!
— Dr. Warrick Stewart, author of Daring Love, drwarrickstewart.com

I'm going to recommend this to adults for their own understanding of what happened to them!
— Louis F. Damis, PhD, ABPP, FASCH

I've known Dr. Hamilton professionally and personally for over a decade now and the results she gets with her integrity, heart, and mission helping both adults and teenagers with severe GI and Autoimmune problems are nothing short of astonishing. I particularly loved the chapter on what not to say to an anxious child which actually could be applied to anyone at any age. Overall, I highly recommend it.

— Elizabeth Bonet, PhD, LMHC

Your book is truly amazing! I honestly can't get enough of it. It is such a relatable and easy read. You have also helped so many of my clients when I send them your podcasts. You are able to be so raw with your own walk and it's so refreshing.

— Dawn Cohen, LCSW, Mom

I'm in tears...Your book is amazing! I think the book was laid out nicely. I like the balance of personal stories and facts/science.

— Melissa, Mom

This is an excellent and insightful book offering a fascinating exploration of the intricate links between trauma, autoimmune disorders, and gut health. The author's engaging writing style makes complex scientific concepts accessible to a general audience, illuminating the powerful mind-body connection that underlies our overall well-being. A particular strength is the focus on the brain-body axis, shedding light on how our neural systems interact with our physical health in profound ways. What sets this book apart is the abundance of practical, actionable advice woven throughout the pages. Rather than simply presenting theories, the author empowers readers with tangible strategies to apply in their own lives. Whether you're seeking to understand your own health journey or support a loved one, this book is an invaluable resource. Its well-researched, yet approachable nature, makes it a must-read for anyone interested in the interplay between trauma, immunity, and gut health. Fantastic work! Loved every word.

— Dr. Faith Galliano Desai, Clinical Psychologist

Empower

Your Child

To Heal

8 Mind-Body Methods to End Anxiety, GI
& Autoimmune Conditions

SKYLER HAMILTON, PHD

FREE Download Available! Join my newsletter and receive the latest on empowering you and your child to heal at drskyler.net.

This book is dedicated to Lakara.

Contents

Foreword   X

A Note From Dr. Skyler   1

Part 1

Laying the Foundation For Healing

1. Why My Child!?!   5
   Your Child's Condition Has a Mind–Body Correlation

2. The Miracle Patient   13
   How "Patient Zero" Provided a Blueprint For Many Others

3. I'm Done (Being Sick)!   23
   My Story, From Wheelchair to Wellness

Part 2

In Your Corner

4. The Hardest Part   32
   Regulating Your Vibes to Avoid Passing on the Stress Contagion

5. What Kind of Parent Are You?   45
   Helicopter, Bulldozer, Avoidant, or Lighthouse?

6. Back In "My Generation"   60
   The Global Rise in Stress, Pressure, and Cyberpsychology

7. Top 10 Things Kids Wish You Knew   69
   Understanding Secondary Gains and Why They Matter

8. The Top 5 Things to Never Say to Your Child With an AI   79
    or GI Condition

Part 3

Becoming a Wellness Warrior

9. Your Child's Healing Phase(s), Part 1   88
    Understanding the Dynamics of the Martyr and the Victim

10. Your Child's Healing Phase(s), Part 2   98
    Moving to the Survivor, Thriver, and Warrior Phases

11. The Privilege of Victimhood   103
    Does Your Child Have the Time and Resources to Feel Sick?

12. Deactivating the Limbic System   109
    Disengaging the Fight Response

13. Landing the Flight Safely   119
    Cultivating Safety When the Mind and Body Want to Flee

14. Melting the Freeze Response   124
    Reframing Threats to Avoid a Mind–Body Shutdown

Part 4

The Balancing Act

15. Family Finances Versus None of Your Business   132

16. The Glass Child Versus the Sick Child   136

17. Are You Trauma-Bonded to Your Child?   142

18. Repurposing the Pain   149

Part 5

The 8 Mind-Body Methods to End Anxiety, GI, and AI Conditions

19. Safety-Based Protocol Steps 1–4   156
    Start With the Scientific Interplay Between Mind and Body

20. Safety-Based Protocol Steps 5–8   160
    Learn to Leverage the Psychology Behind Healing

21.	The Power of Language and Silence Words Can Sabotage or Empower Your Child to Heal	164
22.	The Power of Belief, Finding Flow	167
23.	Mind–Body Panic and Anxiety Hacks	174
Epilogue: Look At You Now!		184
Acknowledgements		186
About the Author		188
Endnotes		191

Foreword

I have known Dr. Hamilton for the past ten years and had the pleasure of collaborating with her on a study that demonstrated the effectiveness of neuroception of safety for the treatment of gut-brain interaction disorders. Working with adolescents and young adults experiencing gastrointestinal and autoimmune disorders has been an area of her expertise long before our collaboration five years ago. This book outlines her vast knowledge of these conditions and the sophisticated neuroscience-based treatment model she has developed.

Disruptions in physiological homeostasis secondary to stress, stress-related disorders, and attachment disruptions have been documented in chronic and recurring conditions such as irritable bowel syndrome, inflammatory colitis/bowel disease, systemic lupus erythematosus, rheumatoid arthritis, Sjogren's syndrome, multiple sclerosis, thyroiditis, and fibromyalgia[1,2,3,4,5,6,7]. Although significant or unusual adverse life events are often identified, more subtle chronic and amorphous stressors can be contributing or etiological factors.

Dr. Hamilton delineates an approach that provides a comprehensive understanding of the complex emotional dynamics underlying the physiological processes contributing to a wide range of somatic conditions that medical interventions alone cannot resolve. Moreover, the often subtle interpersonal and family dynamics that contribute to frequently concealed emotional states are clearly elucidated and translated into strategies that family members and clinicians can apply.

Whereas Polyvagal Theory has provided us with a model to understand the importance of interpersonal safety for promoting health, growth, and restoration, Dr. Hamilton brings us a comprehensive understanding of how to create such an environment for our children. The work of Dr. Stephen Porges[8] has underscored the importance of interpersonal relationships and how they can co-regulate disordered autonomic nervous system activity and restore a physiological state of homeostasis that promotes health and wellness. Through open and genuine personal experiences and clinical case examples, Dr. Hamilton takes us on a journey of self-exploration, insight into our children's minds, and skill development that will foster health, wellness, and success for our children. This book will empower all family members and is a must-read for all parents and clinicians.

— Louis F. Damis, PhD, ABPP, FASCH
Diplomate, American Board of Professional Psychology
Fellow, American Academy of Clinical Health Psychology
Fellow, American Society of Clinical Hypnosis
Fellow, Florida Society of Clinical Hypnosis
Past President, American Society of Clinical Hypnosis
Assistant Professor of Psychology, UCF College of Medicine
Licensed Psychologist
Integrative Health Psychology, PA

A Note From Dr. Skyler

Dear Reader:

The greatest honor a parent can bestow upon me is entrusting their child to my care. It is humbling and the greatest act of trust a parent can give another. This is how I feel as you take your most precious resources in life—your time and your child—to read this book.

Twenty years ago, I lay on the floor of a remote Utah desert screaming out to God, yelling in utter rage and anger, "My life was robbed from me! You robbed me!" After all the anger was released, and half the animal population ran for higher ground, I broke. I broke through the anger and the mountain of sadness that was patiently waiting to come bellowing out from the depths of my soul. I felt relieved. I felt free.

I looked up at God and the clear blue desert sky—by then, I was slightly muddy from my tears drenching the desert sand—and said, "OK, I'll do this! Fine! So be it! I'll suffer. . . But . . . but. . . It has to at least help one person in my lifetime, and then. . . This will all be worth it."

I entered a pact with God that day, vowing a purpose and a life mission. If I only knew that day what He had in store for me as far as suffering at the hands of others, I may have renegotiated the terms. All in all, if this book—my pain, my mistakes, the depths of my suffering over and over, and my Divine healing—have helped one area of your life, it humbles me beyond recognition, and I am abundantly blessed and grateful. Thank you for your time and energy and taking a chance on healing.

Faithfully yours,

Dr. Skyler

Part 1

Laying the Foundation For Healing

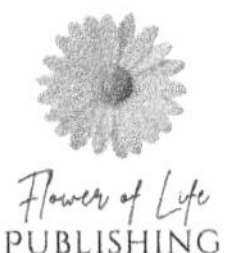

Chapter One

Why My Child!?!

Your Child's Condition Has a Mind–Body Correlation

Finding Dr. Hamilton was nothing short of a miracle for our family. My 16-year-old daughter was struggling with severe anxiety and emetophobia [fear of vomiting], leading to her isolation at home, withdrawing from her magnet school to [do] online schooling, and constantly attempting to avoid all triggers, yet nothing would ease the panic attacks or the fear of having one. Needless to say, I can't begin to describe how much it affected our life as a family. We had to turn everything around to accommodate her condition, from the simple things, such as protecting her from cooking odors, to skipping many trips, outings, and even necessary doctor visits as the mere thought of getting into a car would elicit severe anxiety. As a single mom who has a highly stressful job, it was an additional layer of stress to deal with a condition that I have little to no information about, and we resorted to many psychologists and doctors; we even attempted anxiety medications, to no avail. We were hopeless watching her health decline each day.

Until it all culminated in my daughter's hospitalization on a nasogastric tube after a drastic weight loss and avoidance of most food, and even water, for fear of throwing up.

I was desperate beyond measure at that point, as the previous attempts with psychologists were unsuccessful and my daughter never connected to any of them. I was confused about how to approach the next phase as my daughter was very clear about refusing to be medicated. Then, during the hospital stay, the floor pediatrician mentioned Dr. Hamilton, and everything changed. I checked her website and reached out to her, and she replied immediately. We scheduled a call while my daughter was still in the hospital, and the rest is history. Her compassionate approach, deep understanding, and tailored treatment plan are working wonders.

She connected with my daughter in a way no one else could, providing her with the tools and support she needed to overcome her fears.

Under Dr. Hamilton's care, my daughter's transformation has been remarkable. Her anxiety has significantly decreased, she's gaining weight and strength, she is going out more often, socializing more; she even traveled for six weeks and, most importantly, she's reclaiming her life. Not only that, [Dr. Hamilton] also gave me, as a mom, good advice, and how to deal and connect with my daughter and better understand her condition and expectations. The resources she provided are priceless, and I cannot stop listening to her podcasts. Dr. Hamilton has given us back our daughter, and for that we are eternally grateful.

—Nidale B., Mother

***

Perhaps no other pain compares to a parent dealing with a suffering, sick child with no treatment answers, no apparent causes, and no end in sight. The desperation is palpable. We entertain thoughts like *Will my child live the rest of their life like this? Will they ever be able to go to college with all these medical problems? Will they be able to get married, or have children? Can they ever lead a normal life and be able to take care of themselves?*

I know, because I asked these questions, too. I watched my daughter use a cane to get around, crying in pain, unable to go to school and too sick to have quality friendships. As the medical bills piled up, so did my hopelessness and helplessness. We do what we can for our children, holding them, caring for their needs, and bearing the burdens. I recall feeling so alone, terrified of how I was going to help my daughter, and I cried myself to sleep more times than I care to count. I was alone, isolated, and helpless. No one understood, and no one really cared. Maybe you can relate: It's a horrible feeling.

This—my desire to help other parents not feel as alone as I did, with no answers in sight—was the genesis of this book. There's no "easy" button to push. We parents would gladly trade places with our children as we lose sleep trying to figure it all out. Physicians offer their best treatment for the symptoms, but many times they have to slap a label on a particular condition without knowing where it came from. We enter the trial-and-error phase of treatments, hoping something makes a difference. But, inevitably, nothing does, and we're back to square one: What's wrong with my child?

Most of my patients come from medical doctor referrals, and their parents have reached this tipping point of desperation. Despite their hard work and multiple tests, nothing is working. So, they open their minds to the possibility that there's something else going on, beyond a purely medical explanation. They begin to look outside the box. That's where I come in.

Although I'm a psychotherapist, most of my patients suffer from gastrointestinal (GI) disorders and autoimmune (AI) conditions, which are not widely considered mental health concerns. Yet, they are.

My research, related studies, and experience have pointed to a somewhat obvious answer. Our survival mechanism is designed to prepare us to fight, flee, or freeze, which is helpful if you're facing a tiger, but it's not meant to stay engaged for long periods of time. What does this survival mechanism have to do with your child's condition? Everything.

For example, according to the National Science Foundation, we have roughly 60,000 thoughts a day, and it is that estimated 80 percent of those thoughts are negative, so that equals approximately 48,000 negative thoughts a day. Those 48,000 automatic negative thoughts (aka ANTs) per day create, perpetuate, and foster real and perceived stress, activating the survival part of our brains. Over time, the brain becomes miswired and overtaxed and can be coupled with negative, oftentimes obsessive thoughts, creating and fostering the disease process, more specifically, anxiety, gut health, and AI conditions.

So, the short answer as to why your child is sick is that they are most likely experiencing a chronic limbic response. Medications may be used to try to treat the symptoms, but they will not heal your child. To heal your child, we have to apply a new paradigm largely based on proven, scientific-based psychology.

I've had patients heal from many GI disorders, including chronic constipation, irritable bowel syndrome (IBS), colitis, gastroparesis, Crohn's disease, reflux, rumination disorder, chronic diarrhea, cyclical vomiting, fear of vomiting, gastroesophageal reflux disease, dyspepsia, irritation caused by feeding tubes, neuropathy, mast cell activation syndrome, lupus, thyroid disease, hypervisceral allogeneic abdominal pain and bloating, small-fiber neuropathy, chronic widespread (and abdominal) pain, juvenile arthritis, and debilitating migraines, to name just a few.

Now, I'm going to explain the core concepts and the mind–body systems that underlie my work in healing children from these kinds of conditions. Although you may not need to know exactly how all this works, I've included these explanations so you understand the underlying systems that are at play as we begin to discuss how to empower your child to heal. So, strap yourself in for a few pages.

ANTs, which often develop from psychosocial factors, such as stress, trauma, and neglect, can disrupt communication between the brain and gut. This disruption triggers digestive disorders, referred to as *disorders of gut–brain interaction*.

The body has an incredible ability to maintain homeostasis, largely thanks to its autonomic nervous system (ANS). This ANS is a component of the peripheral nervous system that regulates involuntary physiologic processes, including heart rate, blood pressure, respiration, digestion, and sexual arousal. Now, stick with me here. The ANS has two major divisions, the *parasympathetic* (parasympathetic nervous system [PNS]) and *sympathetic* (sympathetic nervous system [SNS]) branches; these are in part what makes up the limbic region of the brain. The SNS, which we will also refer to as the *limbic system*, is responsible for our survival mechanism—fight, flee, or freeze—responses. The parasympathetic part of the limbic system is responsible for rest and digestion and the freeze response. When the mind is at peace, the body can rest and digest properly. However, if the mind perceives threats, it triggers the limbic system. The PNS and SNS both affect the function of the GI system.[1]

Along with my own research, personal experience, and anecdotal evidence after working with hundreds of patients, a large body of scientific evidence supports the effectiveness of psychological treatments for gut-brain conditions. In our study, a colleague and I focused on increasing the participants' sense of safety. Feelings of being safe and warm were consistently related to reduced abdominal pain and IBS symptoms, but feeling relaxed had no effect on the participants' symptoms. This suggests that one can feel relaxed but not safe. You can have low arousal, or feel your body relax as you begin to fall asleep, but your mind can still be racing. I'm sure the mothers out there can relate to this.

Therefore, lower arousal levels and relaxation are not indicative of feeling safe. Feeling safe is directly linked to the limbic system, which is in charge of our GI and immune systems. In other words, the brain and gut are constantly talking to each other—or perhaps arguing. Also, ANTs jeopardize our internal sense of safety, and is where this journey begins.

To explore even further, the brain has yet another way for the body to trigger the survival mechanism: The brain scans the environment for perceived dangers through a process called *neuroception*. According to a pioneer in this research, Stephen Porges, "Neuroception describes how your brain distinguishes whether situations or people are safe, dangerous or life threatening. Neuroception explains why a baby coos at a caregiver but cries at a stranger, or why a toddler enjoys a parent's embrace but views a hug from a stranger as an assault."[2] The strangers may be safe, and even a loved one likely is safe, but the baby's mind perceives danger. Just because the stranger is a loved one does not mean the baby should not feel frightened. The baby feels unsafe regardless of how you think they should feel. Keep this key concept in mind as we dive deeper into the book, because there is a difference between how our children feel as opposed to how we think they should feel. Two truths can exist simultaneously and still be opposing.

Neuroception, along with emotions, is the link between the mind and the body. Emotions serve as the glue that holds the mind and body together. Neuroception, emotions, and ANTs trigger the limbic system's fight, flee, or freeze response.

Let me give you an application of how this works. When we see a tiger approaching us in the wild, we acknowledge the threat through neuroception. The body jumps into action, releasing adrenaline and cortisol hormones, engaging a response from the limbic system, the part of the brain responsible for keeping us safe by determining whether we should fight, flee, or freeze. These hormones prompt a cascade of changes, quickening our heart rate, sharpening the senses, and pulling resources from the body to enable us to focus on, and react to, the immediate danger. This may include fighting back, fleeing as fast as possible, or, if there's no chance of escape, freezing and hoping the threat passes. When the danger subsides, the body can return to a state of equilibrium and send the excess hormones through the gut for elimination. In other words, our limbic system was never designed to be on constant alert.

In today's society, our neuroception is on heightened alert, always scanning for dangers or perceived threats, like our own thoughts, assignments, deadlines, social media, grades, bills, people-pleasing, fear of displeasing parents, unhealthy attachment styles, and much more. This leads to emotions that confirm for our body that there is a threat, one that is worthy of fear, anger, frustration, and doubt, among other possible emotions.

Therefore, the entire fight-or-flight process starts with what we perceive as a threat. Although we don't have to fear wild tigers, our brain picks up threats from the ever-present news cycle reporting about war, pandemics, financial crises, disease, and death along with myriad topics related to family dynamics, conflicts, social media, the failure to please, fears of failure, shootings, and pressures at school, among many others. There is a continuous level stress coursing through our veins reaching the roughly 25 trillion cells in the human body.

This is what I mean when I refer to the mind–body connection, which has a more scientific name: *psychoneuroimmunology.* This mind–body connection involves the *vagus nerve,* which connects the brain to the gut, playing an important role in maintaining the body's homeostasis and influencing cardiac and GI functions.

So, why is your child sick? Let's recap what we've covered so far: (1) We have ANTs that release emotions, which are the glue (neurochemicals and hormones) that binds the mind to the body, thereby affecting the immune and endocrine systems; (2) neuroception, which detects threats and cues (3) the limbic system's fight, flight, or freeze response; and (4) the vagus nerve, which connects the brain to the gut and helps communicate all these data to the gut as it passes through the heart and various organs on the way down. These four elements, in large part, make up the mind–body connection and are major players in your child's disease process.

Interestingly, the gut has the second highest concentration of neurons after the brain. It's literally the second brain in the body, with the heart being the third.

The environment in the gut is referred to as the *microbiome.* A microbiome is a community of microorganisms, such as fungi, bacteria, and viruses, that helps with digestion, regulation of the immune system, and protection of our bodies from illness or disease, to name a few.[3] The gut microbiota are critical for maintaining health in the immune system. Because gut microbiota and the brain are interconnected in a bidirectional relationship, evidence links anxiety and depressive disorders to disruptions to the community of microbes in the gut. Therefore, ANTs, emotions, neuroception, and an overactive limbic system all disrupt the gut's microbiome community. Plus, the gut provides approximately 95% of the body's "happy hormone," serotonin.[4] So, it's no wonder that when we feel sick to our stomachs, we also feel depressed.

Autoimmune Answers

Research suggests there are more people suffering from AI conditions than heart disease, diabetes, and cancer—combined! With the gut microbiota's profound effects on the immune system, it is not surprising that the gut has been linked to AI diseases. Obviously, the immune system plays a vital role in keeping the body healthy. According to the Autoimmune Association, there are over 100 known AI diseases. Some well-known AI diseases include type 1 diabetes, multiple sclerosis, lupus, rheumatoid arthritis, psoriasis, Crohn's disease, and scleroderma. Symptoms of AI disorders vary according to the type and location of the faulty immune response but may include fatigue, fever, a general ill feeling (malaise), joint pain, and rash. AI diseases can affect almost any part of your body. Treatment for AI diseases has left many in the medical field hapless because of the wide range of symptoms and disparity of possible causes. I hope that by the end of this book you will feel you have answers, explanations, and tools.

Genetic Explanations

Another factor to explore is the epigenetic transmission of trauma that alters genetic expression in children even before they are born. Research has confirmed that adverse childhood experiences may influence the next generations (epigenetics). Epigenetics potentially explains why effects of trauma may endure long after the immediate threat is gone.

Passing down generational stress and trauma to our children is real. For example, adult children, grandchildren, and great-grandchildren of Holocaust survivors are more likely than others to have mood and anxiety disorders, as well as post-traumatic stress disorder (PTSD).[5] Furthermore, many Holocaust offspring also had high cortisol levels—something that we had observed in their parents and grandparents with PTSD.

Therefore, your child's illness could be attributed as far back to their great grandparents' stress, anxiety and other consequences from emotional trauma.

What does this all mean?

There's hope. And, you're not helpless.

If the mind can create so much stress that the body creates illness, then the opposite is also true. The mind can relieve the body of stress that creates wellness by rewiring the contributing factors of anxiety and undoing the tangled gut–brain axis that formed their GI and AI disorders. This is the basis on which the rest of the book is formed and which has helped hundreds of my patients heal their "mysterious" conditions.

When the brain is in a limbic state, the body is in limbo. The body is a physical representation of the mind. So, the answer to solving your sick child's problem(s) is related to rewiring the brain to detect fewer threats; recognizing their ANTS; and creating a new paradigm that harbors safety, peace, and well-being. Therefore, our journey will seek to rewire the subconscious mind and body, to feel safe, heard, and validated so it can maintain proper homeostasis. Because when the mind is at rest, the body will digest.

Chapter Two

The Miracle Patient

"Hello, Dr. Hamilton? I am calling from Arnold Palmer Children's Hospital. I'm Dr. Safder, and we have a very sick 17-year-old female patient.

"OK," I said. "How can I help?"

Dr. Safder, an innovative and compassionate gastroenterology physician, began to explain to me how her patient, Ruthie, has a gastrostomy–jejunostomy (G-J) tube (which sends nutrition directly to the stomach while venting air). Dr. Safder was thinking outside the box of conventional Western medicine because all medical options had been implemented, to no avail. This was Ruthie's last hope. "We need your help as a clinical hypnotherapist," she pleaded. "We don't see any organic reason that would be causing these symptoms. She just can't keep anything down. So, I've heard of your work, and wanted to try an alternative approach."

I had been swimming laps when I got Dr. Safder's call. Over the next hour, I paced back and forth across the pool deck as Dr. Safder gave me a crash course on functional gastrointestinal (GI) disorders. As we spoke, something deep inside my soul knew, just knew, that I could help this child. This same instinct has guided me all these years and has healed my own autoimmune (AI) disease.

That call began my journey to empower children to heal themselves from functional GI and AI disorders. And Ruthie, the struggling teenager, became my Patient Zero. She had been diagnosed with dyspepsia, irritable bowel syndrome (IBS), and severe rumination disorder. When I met her, I saw a young woman who seemed to be decaying. She was malnourished because her body had rejected all different types of feeding tubes. The port from her G-J tube had repeatedly become infected. She had flatlined, nearly dying seven times from sepsis, a serious condition in which the body responds improperly to an infection. She was in and out of consciousness. I was told she had spent more time in the hospital than at home, and her parents were told at one point to have her Last Rites read over her unconscious body. Her family had prayed over her bed, helplessly, countless times. The doctors even prayed, because they had no answers and thought she would never have a typical life—if she survived—let alone a life where she would thrive. Not even Ruthie was sure if she would live or not. Yet, after speaking with her briefly, I could tell she was highly dedicated and motivated to heal. So, for me, half the work was already done based on her belief that healing was possible.

Ruthie had not been able to consume solid foods for more than 3 years without having excruciating, life-debilitating pain that would leave her hospital bound for weeks at a time. She had been sick for more than 5 years. She couldn't even stand the pain of prescribed liquid nutrients when they reached her gut, even with a feeding tube sending them directly into the stomach. She could feel the liquid from the feeding tube with such intense pain that she was forced to stop using a nasogastric (NG) tube. She was compelled to stop eating altogether because of hypervisceral sensitivity to the NG tube, so her doctors inserted the more complex G-J tube, which reached the end of her stomach to avoid the hypersensitivity. With some of the best pediatric GI medical care in the world, no one could seem to find the right medical intervention to help this child. There simply was no medical explanation, effective treatments, or answers. She was in such debilitating, excruciating pain that her life as a typical teen seemed to be over. She spent her days linked up to tubes, at doctors' appointments, or staying in the hospital. She was then placed on the stomach transplant list in a hospital in Miami. This was everyone's last hope, even though her medical team was not sure she would even survive the surgery. If something did not change, Ruthie would die.

My instinct told me I could help Ruthie, and I've since realized we all possess the same instinct. It's a "knowingness" that resides in the place of infinite peace and wisdom we all have access to. But it hides in fear, under the static and the guise of "I'm too busy," or "I can't do that—what if it doesn't work for me?" It hides under stress, work, bills, and autonomic negative thoughts (ANTs). ANTs perpetuate, foster, and nourish disease. ANTs are the nutrients that feed a state of disease, and if those ANTs are nourished enough, feeding on a diet of fears, that state eventually blooms into a full-blown disease. Then, fostered in the right environment of stress and pressure (whether it be external or internal pressures), the disease gets worse. This applies to both adults and children.

During my first, one-on-one meeting with Ruthie, I began to notice there was more going on than physical ailments. Her mind and body were experiencing multiple levels of chronic stress, and her immune system wasn't able to catch up with the constant flow of stress hormones. The next time we met, we dug deeper and identified several sources of stress in her life, and we began crafting an action plan. After the third session with me, her doctor removed Ruthie's G-J tube. By our fifth session, she took her first bite of food in 3 years—peanut butter—and it stayed down with no pain.

Within a month of working together, Ruthie had her first meal in 3 years, at a well-known chicken fast food place. She had been craving their waffle fries for years and wanted those specific fries to celebrate her ability to consume food now. In the years before she had been forced to stop eating because of abdominal pain and IBS symptoms, she had vomited all food, even liquids, immediately after she swallowed them. Yet she did not have an eating disorder.

How did Ruthie go from years of not being able to swallow any food, and being on a stomach transplant list, to eating waffle fries in a fast food restaurant a month later? In short, her three-word treatment plan was this: *(un)freeze, family, and faith.*

Later in the book, I'll describe more about *how* to empower your child to heal, but for now I want to describe the moments that stood out while I witnessed Ruthie's miracle in real time.

When she began to unlock her ANTs, unpack the family skeletons, and discover her sense of self, she admitted, "I don't know who I am outside of my disease." With my help, she was able to unfreeze her frozen limbic response as she spoke her truth and her emotions and perceptions were validated. Slowly, she started to connect with her emotions while realizing it was OK to speak her truth—to tell her parents all the things she wished they knew. The limbic part of the brain is responsible for keeping us safe; this includes activating the fight, flight, or freeze responses. In Ruthie's case, she was in "freeze" mode, a dissociative response that feels like a numbness and disconnected her from her mind and body and an utter disengagement with her emotions. She had been immobilized from prolonged external and internal stressors, and her emotional suffering instructed her mind to "shut off" in certain ways. This is called the *dorsal vagal complex*, and it is a response we will cover in greater detail in Chapter 14. Ruthie's emotional pain manifested as guilt, and over time it became deeply entrenched in her body. From the outside, she looked happy, with lots of friends, a competitive athlete with excellent grades. But she had years of hidden emotional pain, along with two very supportive parents. It is common for children and adolescents to present a brave face to their parents as they suffer in silence. This all became too much for Ruthie, and her brain went into a very adaptive, but eventually maladaptive, response to keep her safe from her own pain.

During our sessions, we began to explore the hidden pain behind her family dynamics, providing her tools she could use to protect herself from their stress contagion and to express her needs and boundaries and disarm her ANTs.

The second ingredient to Ruthie's miracle involved her family, specifically, her parents' willingness to be vulnerable enough to send Ruthie to me and allow her to reveal the proverbial skeletons in the family's closet. The amount of respect and honor I hold for her family is immense. The courage to allow another human to access your worst moments in life and selflessly serve your child is the act of an ideal parent. A parent who is willing to sacrifice their pride and ego, and face their shame and fears, makes for the ideal parent I truly enjoy working with and gently educating. Healing their child was more important to Ruthie's parents than me learning of their family dysfunction. I wish all parents were like this. I could help many more children if all parents had this humility and courage.

Ruthie became my miracle patient, and the reason behind a term I coined: the "Ruthie Ripple Effect," referring to the powerful impact family dynamics (the external environment) have on a child's health. The effect of adverse childhood experiences (ACEs) on health outcomes, including heart disease, diabetes, high blood sugar, and cancer later in adult life, has long been established. Witnessing first hand the ACEs that result from specific family dynamics, ANTs, and the external pressures children face, along with everything else that plays a role in their mental health, is mirrored in a child's body and the disease process. I was not prepared for this in graduate school. It is both awe inspiring and terrifying at the same time.

As we unraveled Ruthie's family's dynamics, and her stressors and pressures, I began to realize the utter sheer power of the gut–brain axis, which is bidirectional and intricately linked to the limbic system as it extends from the esophagus to the rectum. A person's gut can be a direct mirror, reflecting one's thoughts.[1] Research has shown that IBS can be a result of a dysregulated nervous system. Children are directly impacted by their external environment because they have no control over their lives in general (later in this book we will explore the concept of autonomy).

Ruthie taught me that a child's external environment encompasses many things over which they have limited control. Issues like family dynamics, school, sports, grades, friends, performances, dance classes, and social media all create an internalized stressful environment that can foster GI problems. This can lead to thoughts such as, *I'm never good enough. I am not smart enough. I am not skinny enough. Nothing I do is good enough. I can't fail, or my parents will be disappointed in me. I don't deserve this, I'm not worthy of being loved.* However, these are false ANTs and false beliefs. Ruthie became locked into a chronic, long-term frozen immobilization response, which caused her vagus nerve to be flooded over time. The part of the vagus nerve that is affected is called the *dorsal vagal complex,* as mentioned earlier in this chapter. It's a complex, and brilliant, mechanism of the brain that, when in the limbic frozen state, is analogous to playing possum or being immobilized like a deer in the headlights. In this state, the body becomes numb to emotions in order to survive the environment.

Still, something amazing happened. When Ruthie and I dismantled her ANTs and began to unpack the family skeletons, she began to unfreeze.

On a parallel path to deconstructing her freeze state and its family-related causes, we journeyed into a discussion of how Ruthie's faith could play a critical role. In one session, we listened to a specific song, to rewire her mind. While engaging in the music, we both felt a powerful light and energy that literally brought us both to our knees. To this day, that moment still brings tears to my eyes. I will remember forever the moment we were enveloped by a Divine energy so overwhelming it was almost unbearable. From it, she drew her own energy, strength, and courage.

In addition to her faith, we used meditation and hypnosis, a deep understanding of her family dynamics, identifying her ANTs and her secondary gains to help rewire her brain. (I'll go into detail about secondary gains in Chapter 7, but in brief, they are the benefits that often come from being sick.) Music became the subconscious conduit that assisted the process. It started with her stomach growling during a session, her first hunger cue in years! She was so confused, and then remembered, "Wait—this is hunger!?" Her parasympathetic nervous system, the part of the nervous system responsible for rest and digestion, had been engaged in a more adaptive way as she defrosted from her freeze response, understood her false beliefs and pressure, and stepped into the unknown world of trusting her body to heal itself—aka faith. Ruthie embodied all that I feel is an ideal patient, for the following reasons:

- She had an unwavering drive and commitment and wanted to heal.

- Her faith in the Divine, something bigger than herself, carried her.

- Her mind was open to my message that all her suffering and pain will be repurposed into meaning, wisdom, and life lessons.

- She had a willingness to be vulnerable and open about her family dynamics.

- She did her healing work outside of the sessions and worked every day to immobilize her ANTs and protect her peace from external and internal stressors.

- She deactivated her limbic response with the tools I will list later, and she reminded herself hourly and daily that she was safe now.

I can imagine some of you may be thinking, "This would never happen to my kid." Well, frankly, yes; your child has one of these beliefs, or a variant of them, as do my own children. And so did I during my own disease process. GI disorders are a result of a fear of failure, a fear of not being good enough, a fear of losing control. They can result from a fear of disappointing parents. *If I lose control, I will fail,* or *I won't please those I love.* Each of these fears can typically take the form of unexpressed anger and rage and, eventually, self-hate. When the mind tells itself *I hate myself,* the body follows with betrayal.

Ruthie was my Patient Zero for another reason. She created the mold that I later would learn 95% of my patients would fit. She had the following characteristics:

- Inherent overachiever

- Well-behaved child

- Excels academically

- Active in sport(s), in competitive dance, or as a performer (e.g., band)

- People pleaser

Also, typically my patients may have one very supportive parent, and the other parent may either be anxious or even dysfunctional. When I combine these family dynamics with the other attributes from my evaluation, I can formulate a plan that addresses the internal and external stressors that are causing the child's GI or AI disorders. These kids often feel overextended, running on fumes while dealing with internalized fears and pressures. Even if parents insist on them slowing down, these kids won't slow down. This busyness is, in part, why they are sick. Or perhaps they are in a stressful, anxious environment or were simply born anxious. A transmission of anxiety can be absorbed by the child; I'll discuss this later in the book as well in Chapter 4. In modern society, there is simply no time to just be a kid, with free, uncontrolled time to play, explore, laugh, fall, get dirty, walk barefoot on the ground, and climb or swing on trees. This matters. These days, when children do get free time, they sleep, or they scroll on their devices, numbing themselves from reality.

As I began to untangle Ruthie's ANTs, beliefs about her life, her fears, and her family dynamics, it was abundantly clear that her environment (internal and external) fed her thoughts and feelings, and her thoughts and feelings became a direct reflection in her gut. Her gut was the somatic manifestation of her stress and emotions. This is called the *biopsychosocial model* of functional GI disorders, and it refers to the bi-directional communication from the brain to the gut via the vagus nerve.

The vagus nerve is the longest nerve in the body; it travels from the brain to the gut as it innervates and affects the cardiovascular, respiratory, immune, and endocrine systems. Think of it as a direct telephone line from the brain to the gut. Quite literally, this is the mind–body connection. Our thoughts and emotions can affect, and oftentimes dictate, our health. In addition, the gut microbiome (which consists of microorganisms such as bacteria, viruses, protozoa, and fungi) is directly impacted by the mind and body's exposure to prolonged stress, anxiety, and trauma. Our gut produces 95% of our "happy hormones" in the form of what is called *serotonin*.[2] So, when stress hormones disrupt the gut microbiome, the gut is not able to provide sufficient amounts of serotonin. When our physical health deteriorates, our thoughts and feelings of happiness, which are bidirectional and influence AI and GI conditions, are affected. It is incumbent upon us as parents to understand this portion of the disease process. It is critical for us as parents to know the power we hold to help our child heal and to monitor their ANTs, emotional safety and autonomy, and nervous systems. It is this gut–brain relationship, which is underappreciated, along with the internal and external environment in which our children live, that is critical to healing. Parents can help but more often hinder this complex process.

The mind and body work in unison to reach a state of *homeostasis*, or harmony. Too much pressure can elicit the fight, flight, or freeze response. This mind–body relationship is a profoundly complex interconnected system that is deeply interwoven into the AI disease process as well. We will explore this at length and help demystify the processes to empower you to help your child with an AI or GI condition.

Although initially, I knew I could help Ruthie, none of us—her family or medical personnel included—could have imagined she would be so healed 5 years later. She married, and had a child. Now, Ruthie is thriving and living a life she once could only dream of while lying in a hospital bed.

I came to realize Ruthie would serve as a prototype. She cast the mold for hundreds of children I would end up treating. They all share more or less the same characteristics and traits. With Ruthie, my life's purpose, to empower children to heal themselves, began. My journey into the mind–body connection bloomed, and I began to focus on pediatric AI and functional GI conditions. At the time, I didn't fully understand how I had healed myself of multiple sclerosis (see Chapter 3), nor would I have thought I'd be helping many others, including my oldest daughter, using the same techniques and tools I will be teaching you in this book.

As you read this book, occasionally try to see your child through a therapist's eyes. Does your child possess any of the traits I mention? If so, you will want to do as I did, and empower yourself with knowledge and figure out how to help them heal, using this book to guide you.

If you take anything away from this book, let it be this: You don't know your child the way you think you do. I don't want to ruffle your feathers, but I say this with utter confidence on the basis of my work with my own patients and my own two teenage daughters. The things I learned by using the knowledge and tools I am about to teach you will blow your mind. I learned many things when I stopped talking, stopped trying to teach my children lasting life lessons, stopped imparting wisdom, and so on, but instead used the power of silence, and just listened—really *listened* to them—as if I were getting paid to listen to them. What I did not do was defend myself or my actions. In the process, I learned so much. All the knowledge I acquired from listening to them left me sobbing on the closet floor. I treat children, so I have above-average knowledge about their minds, but please know I am not immune to my kids being human; making dumb mistakes on occasion; and having human experiences of pain and suffering, tears, meltdowns, and ANTs. However, I have learned to be comfortable listening to them about my flaws as a parent and as a human and choosing to learn to grow from their feedback. I trust my kids enough to ask them to be vulnerable and real with me. I trust them enough to tell me the truth about how they feel. I get rid of my ego (learned to not defend myself) and listen. I may not always agree with my kids, but I hear them. Creating emotional safety has played a critical role in one of my children healing from her AI condition, going from a walking cane to wearing 70s platform shoes in a year.

When you start this process and get to the heart of your children's needs, their vulnerability and their ANTs, you will learn so much about your child. It will be a huge "A-HA!" "Wow!", and "OUCH!" moment. Until that moment happens, you will remain as clueless as I once was. The more you repeat this process, the less painful it gets, and over time you will master this process and build a bond you would never have imagined was possible! Your child will feel emotionally safe, and this will begin to regulate their nervous system. Emotion regulation has a direct impact on their mental and physical health.

I spend hours a day listening to kids tell me what they wish their parents knew about but are too scared to tell them. I get permission once in awhile from a patient to tell their parents how they feel. Parents get defensive, slam the pen and paper down, yell at their kid, and, even worse, give their child the silent treatment, or walk away in anger, even financially cutting them off. This all hurts the child even more. In the worst cases, the child is forbidden to go to therapy, because I now know all family secrets as the ANTs came marching out of the subconscious mind. One hundred percent of the time, the child gets sicker if their emotions and experiences are not received in an emotionally safe manner. I spend hours preparing parents to receive this feedback to even get to that point to where the child feels safe enough to trust their parent won't react in a harsh or defensive way. And *boom*, they fail in that moment, and the child's trust is gone.

This book will help alleviate the shame or embarrassment of what your kids think and feel because you get to avoid learning this information in front of your kid's therapist. This book will summarize thousands of hours of therapy for you. So, as a mom of a child healing from an AI diagnosis, my mom advice, backed with my clinical education, is this: The more emotional nourishment, safety, and especially autonomy, you provide for your child, the more they will realize that they have the power within themselves to heal. Remember, you are raising an adult, not raising a child. No one of a healthy mindset wants to marry a man-child or a helpless damsel in distress. A parent's job is to raise an emotionally safe human while they are under their care of being a child who is transforming into an adult.

Little did I know at the time that Ruthie would reveal my life's purpose and journey to empower children to heal themselves.

Hang on. It's about to get good.

I'm Done (Being Sick)!

MY STORY, FROM WHEELCHAIR TO WELLNESS

I just wanted to be loved. And I knew how to get that love—even as a 5-year-old tomboy who'd rather climb trees than play with dolls. Unfortunately, my mother wanted me to fit her paradigm of a pretty little girl. I learned that, the hard way.

One Sunday, she fixed my hair in pigtails and dressed me up in my Sunday best. While waiting for her, I went outside to play. When it was time to jump in the car, my mom noticed that I'd scuffed my dress with dirt, and her face transformed into an angry frown.

"You're so dirty!" She yelled from the front seat. "How could you do that?" I couldn't relate to the outburst, so I just stayed silent. As we entered onto the road, she pulled over and told me to get out of the car. "Just GO HOME!" She yelled.

She pulled over in front of our neighbor's house. I knocked on the door. A friendly woman answered. "Hello darlin'," she said in a soft tone. "What are you doing here?"

"Hi," I said sheepishly. "Uh, my mom told me to get out of the car."

"Oh dear," she said. "C'mon in and let's talk." She made me a sandwich and brought a glass of milk. I couldn't figure out why she was being so nice to me, but it felt nice. She called my house and left a message. Eventually, my mom showed up to bring me home.

That was when I started to figure out that, to be loved, I need to look and act a certain way. For my mom, I need to look like a pretty little girl. For others, I needed to look injured and helpless.

At school, a few years later, I fell hard and suffered a concussion. As I waited in the nurse's office for my mom, I got all kinds of loving attention. "Does your head hurt? Do you feel sick to your stomach? Can I get you a juice box?" the nurse asked while stroking my head softly. It felt nice. When my mom arrived, she held me like a precious doll, too.

Uh-huh, this is how you get love. My subconscious seemed to instill this thought in my beliefs. Throughout elementary school, I'd fake injuries, stomachaches, and other maladies so I could experience my mom's nurturing side. I felt worthy, even if I was cheating the system, feigning a physical ailment to obtain nurturing—or what I now call the *secondary gain*. Throughout my childhood, however, those fake conditions started to appear as real, and I was loving it.

***

Strapping on the gloves and whaling away at a punching bag became my new favorite passion. As a 27-year-old training at what used to be Sugar Ray Leonard's gym with the famous boxing referee Richard Steele, I started to get quite accomplished at this brutal sport—so much so that I decided to become a professional boxer.

I trained relentlessly for hours, while keeping my marriage and education afloat. I was wonderfully, physically fit and able to defend myself with my own two fists. One evening, after a particularly hard 4-hour workout, I fell over as my body shook with uncontrollable tremors. I was having what felt like a seizure that featured violent convulsions. Pain coursed through my veins as I rattled on the floor. I couldn't do anything about it. While sobbing as I lay there, I'd lost control over my body as my muscles seized.

"Honey, honey!" my husband shouted. "Can you hear me? Are you OK?"

Although my brain tried to form a sentence, the words could not surface into anything intelligible. Aphasia settled in. My husband was also at a loss for words. He lifted me up in a panic, helped me to the car, and off to the emergency room we went. Upon arrival, I was admitted immediately, and the testing began while I floated in and out of consciousness. I heard the medical staff debate about whether or not I should go to the intensive care unit. I'm not sure where I landed, but I heard someone say I "looked anemic," and the blood test revealed that my iron levels were critically low. Despite my thrashing, I felt a needle pierce my arm, and they hooked me up to intravenous bags of blood. It took two bags of blood to get me to normal levels. Hours later, I began to gain awareness and could speak. The nurses quickly arranged for a doctor to visit me at my bedside.

"Hello, Skyler," the doctor said, walking into my room at a small hospital in St. George, Utah. "I'm Dr. Jones, the resident neurologist here. Can you understand me?"

I nodded.

Then, in a condescending tone, he told me to "Just stop it, you fucking little girl. Stop faking your tremors."

What? I thought, as I was so shocked I didn't know what to say. *Was I faking it?*

"I can see you're a cutter because there's no way you could have lost this much blood and still be walking, let alone boxing," he said with certainty and an air of disregard. "I don't see anything in your blood that would cause this reaction, so I think there's a mental illness going on, which requires a therapist, not a neurologist."

Wait, what? I couldn't believe what I was hearing. *He thinks I'm crazy.* He made a few notes and left the room as quickly as he arrived. Enraged, I demanded that a nurse examine every inch of my body to record that I was NOT a cutter.

This doctor made me question every fiber of my existence, and I felt ashamed, embarrassed, burdensome, and crazy. After all, I had faked illness in the past, but this time I was just along for the ride, completely unable to control my body. I decided to report him to the hospital authorities, and I demanded to be reassigned to a new doctor. The first time I met the new doctor, she seemed very attentive and concerned. "I have some news for you Skyler," she said compassionately. "We discovered you have *oligodendrocytes* in your spinal fluid; there's swelling in your brain and lesions on your optic nerve, brain, and spine."

"Finally, we're getting somewhere," I said. "Thank you Doctor. What does this mean?"

"This is a rather clear-cut case, I'm afraid," she paused. "You have multiple sclerosis [MS]. Additionally, anemia is a common trait of autoimmune and gastrointestinal issues. It's also a sign that you're pushing the limits with your lifestyle. We're going to administer some steroids and monitor your condition for the next few days."

With that, my life would be forever altered.

There was no prognosis for a "normal life," considering how rapidly the disease was progressing. Bound to a hospital bed, I was forced to sit and face the fact that I was physically, mentally, and emotionally withering away. Utterly terrified, I could not accept that this was my life. My dreams for a future full of travel, having a family, and pursuing a nursing career were now hopeless. I wondered if my husband would leave me. I felt robbed and betrayed by my own body. I loathed what I'd become: a meaningless blob that would require special handling the rest of my life. My world, as I knew it, was shattered.

"I wish my mom was here," I told my husband.

He noticed me fading into obscurity, so he did what he could and called my mom to ask her to make the drive from Arizona. This all-too-familiar rescue mission was set into place so I could feel nurtured by my mother.

A few days later, she arrived. She entered the room while I was surrounded by my husband and my boss, who was the kindest nurse I'd ever known, second only to my sister. While I had trained to become a nurse practitioner, I worked for my boss at a nearby hospital. She was attentive, holding my hand, bringing me water, tending to me. She made me feel warm and loved.

Wearing a big smile, my mother greeted everyone, as if she were entering a birthday party. The mood in the room, however, was more serious. "Hi Sweetie," she said as she nodded in my direction. "I stopped on the way to pick up some pajamas for you." She went on about her trip, the traffic, where she had eaten, and other details about her drive. She discussed everything except her child lying right in front of her. The nurses glared awkwardly at her as the room thickened with tension.

My boss interrupted and said, "Maybe we should focus on Skyler right now."

"Oh, yes, how are you doing?" She asked without giving me a chance to reply. "I'm so sorry you are here. I got you some pajamas. I wasn't sure what you wanted to wear, but I knew you wouldn't want to wear a hospital gown, so I think you will like these."

I craved my mother's authentic attention. I needed her to hold my head, tell me she's there for me, that she'll get answers, bring food, and listen to my fears. Instead, she unknowingly neglected my unspoken needs and droned on. It was clear that she didn't have the understanding to show love the way I so deeply craved. Sure, the pajamas were nice, but maybe she, too, thought I was faking it?

She loved me so much and was trying to show me that, with the well-intended pajamas, but her message misfired: She seemed to be trying to fix the "problem." This is a theme you will see throughout the book with respect to well-intended, loving parents. In the midst of the illness, all I wanted was to be held, feel safe, and cry. No one knew what to say, or how to act, including my mom. Having a sick child leaves a mother, at any age, helpless.

After a few weeks, I was released, embarking on a new wheelchair-bound, half-blind journey. The daily struggles turned into a new lifestyle. My husband did leave me after sharing the birth of two children. As a single parent, I began working as a teacher.

My determination to find a treatment or cure to my condition never relented. My doctor suggested I try a new class of medication called a sphingosine 1-phosphate receptor modulator drug, Gilenya, to support a Phase 4 clinical trial. Willing to try virtually anything, I began treatment. Unfortunately, a few days later, I stopped breathing and was taken via ambulance, unconscious, to the emergency room. In a blur, I recall hearing the sirens wail and hearing the words "We're losing her. . . . Bag her!"

Inside my mind, I tried to form the words, "NO! You're not losing me. I'm right here. Do not bag me!" I started getting angry as I heard them scrambling to keep me breathing. As I heard arguments about whether or not to keep fighting to bag me or not, I manage to say my children's names in my head: "Ella. Lily." *You're not breathing, Skyler*, I told myself. *You've got to breathe*. Then, blackness.

I woke up a few hours later in the triage room, with my hand being held by my kids' dad, who was sobbing. *I must have breathed*, I thought.

Turns out, I had experienced respiratory distress from the Gilenya that nearly cost me my life.

A short hospital stay to balance out my system ensued. I then was released to recover at home. The kids' dad had to return to his work, which was over an hour away. With two babies under the age of 2, I needed help managing all the day-to-day tasks, so I called my mom.

"Can you come watch the babies for me please, Mom? I just got out of the hospital again because I had a bad reaction to a drug. I stopped breathing and nearly died. Now, I'm home and need to rest. Would you come for a few days until I feel better?" Of course, as in the old days, I hoped she would provide some loving care, too.

"Oh honey, I'm sorry; I can't," she said. "I am busy. We are skydiving today."

My heart sank. I would have to handle this on my own.

A week or so went by, and I hadn't heard from my brother. He would obviously care to know about my situation, I figured. I called my mom and broke the silence that had existed between us since my near-death experience, "Hey, Mom, I haven't heard from Tony. Did you tell him I almost died?"

"Oh, honey," she said "He is so busy with work. I never get a chance to sit and talk with him."

After a short conversation, I hung up. I hit the wall of rejection. I couldn't bear anymore, and I reached a defining moment.

"I'M DONE!" I shouted. *Done, done, done*, I thought. I finally realized that what I wanted, and needed—even in near-death, I would not get: to feel important enough for someone to care. I drew an invisible line of demarcation in the sand of my suffering. I decided, *This is my last day of being sick.* I was going to heal myself. I *had* to figure this out on my own. I was on a mission to heal. No one was coming.

***

Now, 30 years later, I have the benefit of hindsight, a fundamental understanding of neuroscience, a PhD, and experience working with hundreds of pediatric patients. I understand what I was doing back in those difficult days, and what kids around the globe are experiencing. There are a message and a map to healing hidden under all the pain, the symptoms, and the tears. And, more important, we *all* have tools to unlock and unblock this pain and allow the body to heal itself. The body is designed to heal, but if the naturally restorative processes are obstructed by neurobiological programming from an early age, it cannot do so. Being sick can deliver rewards, secondary gains that create neural pathways that install a reward system. Sickness can lead to feeling freedom from life's pressures. Even though children cry and experience pain, there is a secondary gain being set up in the back stage of the subconscious mind.

My secondary gain started early, when I noticed I could get my mother's attention when I was sick, or faking it. I hold no fault for her, only pure love and acceptance; this was all simply just a part of my journey. I had wired my brain to believe I could gain nurturing love from being sick. Then, my mind began to create illness in my body without me realizing it. Eventually, my body believed my thoughts, which led to a diagnosis of MS and near-death.

I've also learned that physicians and medical personnel have immense power—not necessarily with their diagnoses or treatments, but with their WORDS. Because we respect what they do and say, their words feed our conscious and subconscious minds to determine if we continue to get sicker or heal. In my case, both the secondary gains, and experience with the dreadful neurologist, collided to create the perfect storm to deteriorate.

Now, this is not the case for everyone. This is my story, and my secondary gains. However, there are other secondary gains. There are so many that I had to write this book, because kids get sicker to secretly avoid life's pressures. Children desire parental approval, and they can literally worry themselves sick trying to prove they are worthy, that they are not a disappointment. In turn, they exhaust themselves trying to overachieve; they often end up running on fumes. This leads to living with repressed anger, a sense of foreboding, and worries, which depletes their immune system.

These are the three main themes I see when kids are sick:

- a desire for nurturing and focused attention,

- avoidance of immense amounts of perceived pressure, and

- highly anxious parents and/or dysfunctional family dynamics.

Now, before you go and tell your kid "It's in your head," wait. That will make it 1,000 times worse, I promise. I have the map to help you identify what secondary gain your child may be seeking and how to meet that need. This will deactivate their overstimulated limbic system, which will exacerbate autoimmune and gastrointestinal conditions. In the pages that follow, I'll explain the power of silence and of fostering safety and autonomy to empower your children to heal.

Because if we can "think" and "believe" ourselves into feeling worse, couldn't we "think" and "believe" our way to wellness?

Part 2

In Your Corner

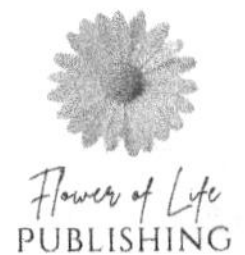

Flower of Life
PUBLISHING

Chapter Four

The Hardest Part

"Honey, I have to talk to you," the dad says to his wife. "Stay calm; there is something I have to tell you: I lost my job today. But it will be OK, I promise. I'll find something as fast as possible."

"WHAT?" The mom responds hysterically, as their daughter eavesdrops from behind the door. "How are we going to pay the mortgage? What will we do about health insurance? Does this mean we can't send our daughter to dance class? Am I going to have to get a job?"

As this hypothetical story unfolds, you can imagine how the anxiety increases over time. Now, imagine what the daughter feels like. From shattered perceptions of her father being a "success," to anticipating the shame she will feel when she tells her dance mates they "can't afford the class," her anxiety must be sky high. Even deeper, the daughter may take on a belief that she will also be a failure.

This is called *stress contagion*, and it feeds illness in ourselves and our children. This contagion includes stress plus all the other emotions we humans experience such as anger, joy, sadness, worry, rage, and fear, to name a few.

Perhaps it's no wonder I get the same answer when I ask each pediatric patient, "If you had one magical wish when you wake up tomorrow morning, and it would come true, what is the one thing you wish you could change in your life?" Surprisingly, it's not that their illness will go away, that they will feel better, that their schoolwork will get easier, or that they will get a new puppy. Instead, the most common answer is, "I wish my parents weren't so stressed out." Clinically speaking, they are pointing out the emotional contagion in the house, the parents' emotional dysregulation—or their "vibes."

Recent research indicates that children with high levels of empathy may experience higher levels of stress-induced physical inflammation and poorer health outcomes when exposed to parental conflict. This study suggested that although empathy is generally a positive trait, in certain environments it can also make children more vulnerable to stress-related health issues.[1]

Another recent study showed that the number one indicator of a child's happiness is the mother's level of happiness.[2]

How is it possible to "catch" the emotions of others? Humans naturally (and unconsciously) mimic the behaviors, posture, and facial expressions of those whom they spend a lot of time around. Over the past decade, science has revealed how our brains are hard wired for emotional contagion.[3] Emotions spread via a wireless network of *mirror neurons*, which are tiny parts of the brain that allow us to empathize with others and understand what they're feeling. When you see someone yawn, mirror neurons can activate, making you yawn. Your brain picks up the fatigue, or joy, response of someone sitting on the other side of the room. But it's not just smiles and yawns that spread. We can also pick up negativity, stress, and uncertainty, much like secondhand smoke.

Not only do emotions get transferred through mirror neurons, but also cortisol (a stress hormone) particles from stress can seep out of the skin, linger in the air, and be absorbed into another human's skin and then into the bloodstream.[4] Let that sink in for a moment, no pun intended. Your cortisol is entering your child's bloodstream (and others around you). According to the latest research on stress contagions, your energy and your stress levels are literally contagious.[5]

Researchers Howard Friedman and Ronald Riggio from the University of California, Riverside, found that if someone in your visual field is anxious and highly expressive—either verbally or nonverbally—there's a high likelihood you'll experience those emotions as well, and this will negatively affect your brain's performance.[6]

Observing someone who is stressed—especially a coworker or family member—can have an immediate effect upon our own nervous systems. A separate group of researchers found that 26% of people showed elevated levels of cortisol just by observing someone who was stressed.[7] Secondhand stress is much more contagious from a romantic partner (40%) than from a stranger.[8]

According to Heidi Hanna, a Fellow at the American Institute of Stress and author of the book *Stressaholic*, secondhand stress is a result of our hard-wired ability to perceive potential threats in our environment: "Most people have experienced spending time with someone who triggers a stress response just by walking in the door. This can be a conditioned response from previous interactions, but may also be an energetic communication delivered by very gentle shifts in bio-mechanical rhythms such as heart rate or breath rate."[9] The cues that cause secondhand stress can be very subtle changes in the people around us at work, yet they can have huge impacts.

In fact, you don't have to see or hear someone to pick up their stress; you can also smell them. New research shows that stress causes people to sweat special stress hormones, which are picked up by the olfactory senses of others.[10] Your brain can even detect whether these "alarm pheromones" were released because of low stress or high stress. Negativity and stress can literally waft into your cubicle.

As research has become more sophisticated, we now know that the negativity we "catch" from others can also affect every single business and educational outcome we can track. Most recently, stress has been shown to affect us down to a cellular level, even shortening our life span.[11, 12]

To summarize, there are at least five ways stress is contagious, especially for highly empathic people: via (1) mirror neurons, (2) cortisol contagion by means of the bloodstream, (3) visual cues, (4) energetic communication through bio-metric rhythms, and (5) smell. So, self-regulating our own stress and emotions is the highest form of love for our children. If we, as parents, can find better ways to cope with our stress and manage our emotions, our children's anxiety levels decrease, which decreases their risk of developing chronic stress-related diseases.

In the Same Boat as You

Helping your child heal begins with becoming aware you are most likely stressed, and your child (and others) can literally catch this stress from you. It's the Ruthie Ripple Effect (see Chapter 1), and it can negatively affect everyone around you. Over prolonged periods of time, this contributes to your child's mental health and disease process. Think of all the times we have come home from a long day at work or have gotten stressed over medical bills or the sheer constant struggling of balancing life with a sick child. It's overwhelming, and no one else understands. It's like a club we never signed up for.

I am in the same boat as you all: the tears, meltdowns and crying on the bathroom floor, feeling helpless, scared, drowning in medical bills, and all those overwhelming fears of the unknown. My daughter was diagnosed at age 14 with juvenile ankylosing spondylitis, which is arthritis of the spine and hips. She became symptomatic after a few bouts with COVID-19 and was gratefully, quickly diagnosed because we have an amazing pediatrician who suspected it was an autoimmune condition as a result of the COVID-19 vaccine coupled with the viral exposures.

I had ever-present ruminating thoughts: *What will her life look like? Will she end up in a wheelchair, like me? Will she be able to carry a child?* She was withering away to skin and bones and had to use a walker to get around. She was always crying and in so much pain. She couldn't go to school, because it was too painful to walk the halls and sit at a hard school desk. She suffered from bad brain fog, so she couldn't follow basic conversations, let alone complete complex math equations. She missed going out with her sister, and her friends, because all she ever wanted to do was sleep and cry. It is devastating to witness a once-vibrant, healthy, balanced child become consumed by disease. It's an extreme form of sheer helplessness as a parent to hear, over and over, from physicians that there is nothing they can do but manage the symptoms and try to keep them from getting worse. It was so frustrating to be on THIS side of the table.

I asked about mind–body therapy, or mind–body options, and the doctors told us to do yoga. That is great, but I needed someone like me to treat my child. Ethically, I'm not supposed to treat family, plus I would get the biggest eye roll and gasp of absurdity if I ever even mentioned it to my daughters. No matter how much I reminded her that "Hey, I get paid for this advice," they still snickered at me with the all-too-familiar "Yah . . . OK, Mom." So, I was just as helpless as every other parent out there. Then, I realized, I am in the same boat as millions of parents. BUT—I have the oars! I can navigate this journey.

My life seemed like a clown's juggling act as I managed a busy private practice, being a single mother of two teen girls, and caring for one horse and one dog. I had four souls under my care, as well as 40 patients depending on me to show up at my best weekly, yet I couldn't have been more alone. I had no supportive partner and no family close by. I couldn't break; too many people depend on me being *their* pillar. So, like millions out there, I understand feeling like the weight of the world is on your shoulders. This is when I realized that there was the one major element I have control over: ME! I can control my stress level and keep it away from my children. I can navigate all of this behind the scenes and still help my daughter without "treating" her. It was a huge "A-ha" moment. A surge of self-efficacy flooded my brain because I knew I had the ability as a human, as a mom, to effect positive change. If anyone is equipped to handle a chronically ill child, and help that child heal, it's me.

This is what I am going to pass on and teach you. Helping your child heal begins with *you*. Unfortunately, it's also the hardest part.

Regulating Your Own Vibes

If your child is willing, please get them a therapist if you don't already have one. It takes a village to raise a child, and we don't live in villages anymore. Helpful tip: Have them pick the therapist (or at least involve them in the selection process). Try not to pick the therapist for them, because success rates increase if they feel bonded to the therapist.[13]

Like anyone, after a 12-hour work day I am not immune to feeling that I have no bandwidth left to be a mom, chef, taxi driver, dog walker, a mommy therapist (not clinically, just listening daily who is dating whom, and the daily emotional download with two children); meet everyone's needs; and ensure my own self-care, such as walking, mediation, and so on. Time seems to never be on our side when we are in the thick of parenthood. With all we have going on in life, I can relate to the resistance of being told "You have to take care of yourself." Prioritizing yourself is probably the last thing on your plate right now. Before you blow off this book, or this chapter, please know that empowering your child to heal begins with modeling this behavior yourself.

I will shepherd you on how to help your child, but first, we parents must humbly accept we're probably overly stressed. For the greater benefit of your child and their health, and to limit the spread of stress contagion, self-care must be a top priority. I am going to give you tools and real-world advice based on my expertise and experience, but if you do not model healthy self-care then none of it will work. You hold immense power in either helping your child feel better or contributing to their disease process. This is a choice you can make and commit to and have control over. If you are done feeling helpless, this process starts with helping yourself.

Having the oars and confidence to navigate my family through this, I committed to regulating my own vibes as my new full-time job—managing me better so I am *not* what my patients tell me their parents are. When I'm stressed out, my children don't want to be around me: They scatter like cockroaches when I walk into a room and dread hearing the car pull into the driveway. Knowing that emotional contagion is very real, this is what I want to avoid.

I'm confident you can relate. Imagine you have a very difficult boss or coworker, family member, room mom, or teacher who rubs you the wrong way with their energy, mood, and words. Now, how much of that affects you the rest of the day? It's no wonder our children eventually feel it, too. Emotions, and stress in particular, are highly contagious because we are empathic beings. We feel others' pain. It's been on the rise in our society ever since that tragic day in New York that resulted in what I call *The 9/11 Effect*. I'll address that later in the book.

When assessing a patient, I look for the stress inside of them and how much of that stress they are catching from someone else. More than half of the time, the source of the child's stress is not their own inherent pressures. Instead, they have caught the stress contagion from their own parent's anxious vibes.

As we age, empathy gets harder. But kids don't have the same hardened hearts and minds as many adults do, and are therefore they are very empathic. The way I learn about a child's source of stress is by gaining a baseline of how the child responds to potential or imagined stressful situations as we engage in what they believe are casual conversations. If they have high self-efficacy or an ability to gain self-efficacy and increase their confidence levels, then typically they have been taking on stress shared by one or both of their parents. Although there is a genetic component to how well we deal with stress, we can also learn how NOT to pass anxiety or depression down to our children.

Once I discover that the source of the child's stress is coming from the parents, I teach the child mental survival skills that protect their mind and body from their environment. Most of the time, I find the children are actually very chill. For example, one coping skill is for the child to imagine they are bubble-wrapped or have a Wonder Woman shield or a protective force field surrounding them. This mental imagery is used to prevent scary situations from entering their mind and body so they can remain centered in peace or their own vibe. Sometimes, I suggest they put music on, as if it's signaling the force field to go up so they can stay in their own zone. So many cases of gastrointestinal conditions are resolved by using this trick. In later chapters, I share many more strategies for parents and their sick children.

But I want to set the stage here. We as parents must recognize that the way we act, feel, and speak all affect our children's health. Even the way we move, do the dishes, drive the car, get the groceries, and converse with our spouse or partner, influence the environment our children must live with. They are watching! They are aware of our mood and temperament, even if they don't express how they feel. Please do not feel like I'm pointing a finger at you, blaming you for your child's illness. I know that dealing with a sick child can be an emotionally painful experience for parents. Don't avoid it, or fear the pain, and don't stuff it away. Recognize it, and improve—and your child will, too.

I do, however, want to emphasize how big a role we parents play with empowering our children to heal. Besides, I'm with you. I have flaws and am a constant work in progress because that comes with the parenting territory. The main difference between you and me is that this is my profession and my life's work, which I've studied at length to achieve. I'm writing this from two unique perspectives. The first is as a psychotherapist who specializes in somatic disorders and chronic illnesses. I've studied this topic for 20 years, authored research papers, and observed these conditions time and again with patients and parents. My second perspective is as a person who was once diagnosed with multiple sclerosis, and my family dynamics were major players in this.

Four Ways to Boost Your Emotional Immune System

How can we prevent spreading bad vibes while building natural immunity to secondhand stress in our children? The short answer is to mirror positive vibes. In the following sections, I describe my top four ways to boost your, and your child's, emotional immune system.

1—Protect Your Peace

"Protect my peace" is one of my personal mantras. Not many things in life are more important to me than protecting my peace. I may not always have it, but once I get it back it's my job to keep it and protect it for my own health and for those I love. Inner peace is not a new concept. Still, it's easy to read, yet hard to practice. By now you can guess that the first naturally drawn conclusion is to cultivate and protect your inner peace. Just as stress begets stress, peace begets peace.

I now suggest a few strategies to protect your peace.

Avoid People Who Are Stressed

Because we can catch stress through contagion from others, stress that affects our mood and related actions, we can help ourselves and children by avoiding others who are stressed. Because parents set the tone at home, we have to be mindful how we use our most precious commodity—energy—and who we spend our time with. This includes reading the news, perusing negative social media, gossiping, complaining about life, and bringing work home. Follow this guideline: Avoid the Four C's: complaining, comparing, criticizing, and condemning. Your child's nervous system will thank you, and they will catch your peaceful vibes.

Shield Yourself in a Cake Dome

I teach my patients to imagine they are living under a force field, protected from others' energy or vibrations. To help them visualize this, I describe it as a glass cake dome. Personally, I've learned to use this tool when hearing patients recall traumatic memories so that I can stay in a safe space and not be impacted by their trauma and so I can operate from a clinical platform. I have empathy, but I don't get caught in their pain.

I'll never forget how painful my work could be until I learned this tool. I used to work with people who had endured severe, unimaginable trauma. I would come home from work sobbing and emotionally drained from all the pain until I began to protect my peace bubble. Now, if someone in my vicinity—say, at the grocery store or in another public venue—is having a "freak out," I imagine going quietly under my cake dome to avoid catching their bad ju-ju. This may sound silly, but every patient I teach this reports back what a huge difference this technique makes. Interestingly, children on the spectrum seem to do the best with this tool. Kids and young adults LOVE this method. As mentioned earlier, some imagine being encased in bubble wrap, or inside a large, clear blow-up ball, or a Wonder Woman shield. The invisibility cloak from the Harry Potter books is a very popular one. There are many creative ways to ask your child, even a young adult, how they would like to protect themselves using their imagination to shield themselves from energy they feel is too intense. My own younger daughter used this once after I got upset with her. I said, "Why are you not reacting? I am very upset with you!" She responded, "I'm not catching your bad vibes, Mom; *you* taught me this." I didn't know whether to be proud of her or angrier.

Tune In So You Can Tune Out

Music is the fastest way to recalibrate your internal state of being. Music is vibrational, and vibrations influence us. Music can reduce stress and increase dopamine levels. A slow, steady rhythm (60–80 beats per minute, the resting heart rate) may provide stress reduction by altering body rhythms and bringing back a sense of peace. Scientists believe that the 8-minute song "Weightless" by Marconi Union is particularly effective in reducing stress and anxiety.[14] Listening to this song lowers blood pressure and heart rate and creates a state of peace.[15]

Healing beat music may be used as a treatment method to relieve stress in daily life contexts. I used music to rewire my brain as I was healing, and I use music daily to dance, raise my energy levels, or, if I'm stressed, to create peace. I love using the power of music to help rewire the brain. I have my patients create a wellness playlist, and we go over the lyrics in each song to ensure they promote a sense of wellness.

Music was a very large part of healing for my very first patient, Ruthie (see Chapter 1). She wanted to use faith-based music during our sessions, and she listened in her free time as well. It was as we were listening to her favorite song that we watched a miracle occur in real time as she took her first bite of food in years. She felt the power of the words, used her strong belief in faith, and trusted that her body could welcome, accept, and retain nutrients.

The lyrics you sing and listen to get wired into the brain; thus, music is among one of the top ways to create neuroplasticity. Because music is oftentimes tied to emotion, it becomes deeply wired in the brain. Think of this as being like snow tracks: music makes the snow tracks even deeper. How you think is how you feel, how you feel is how you behave, and how you behave creates habits. Here is an interesting fact: When I conduct an intake session with a patient who has depression, I have them show me their playlist, and if it contains negative language or messages that is one of the first changes we make.

Music was the first healing tool my older daughter used. Music became one of the single biggest catalysts that helped her find her stride and use the power of the mind to create a sense of wellness in her body through music. She calls her playlist her "happy playlist."

Water Does the Mind and Body Good

Listening to water sounds is beneficial as well. Studies suggest that natural sounds, like running water, have a stress-reducing effect that changes the endocrine and the autonomic nervous systems.[16] This implies that listening to natural sounds may be a simple and easily accessible intervention that is capable of positively affecting the stress systems. In addition, routine immersion bathing appears to be more beneficial to one's mental and physical health than routine showers. Taking a warm bath to obtain more immediate stress relief creates inhibition of the sympathetic nerves and stimulation of the parasympathetic nerves, creating an internal sense of peace. Water has amazing healing benefits and promotes stress reduction. Also, recent science is pointing to the wide range of benefits from cold water exposure or cold plunges.[17] I discuss this further later in the book.

Give Yourself a Self-Esteem Boost

One of the greatest buffers against picking up others' stress is nurturing a healthy self-esteem. The higher your self-esteem is, the less anxiety you will have, and the more likely it is that you will feel that you can deal with whatever situation you face. If you are finding yourself at risk of being impacted by others' moods, stop or pull away for an auto-correct moment. Remind yourself that you can handle anything that comes your way. *You have a 100% survival rate.* There are life situations that come and go, and there is life. The life situation will pass and you can remind yourself, "You got this." Exercise is also one of the best ways to build self-esteem because, through endorphins, your brain records a victory for the effort every time you exercise. So, if you didn't already have a doctor telling you to exercise your body, now you have one telling you that it will help your mind, too.

2—Inoculate Yourself With Good Vibes

The second way to boost your emotional immune system is by taking the proactive, preventative measure of inoculating yourself with a good vibe vaccine. For example, before entering the daily rat race the first thing we can do is think of three things we are grateful for that day. I suggest getting into the practice of inoculating yourself immediately after waking up, as you are coming to terms with your consciousness. This sets your intent and mindset for the day. Try answering any or all of the following in a journal entry:

- How can I create peace today?

- What great things will I experience today?

- How can I surrender to my day with grace and resilience?

A part of the brain called the *reticular activating system* will scan your environment all day long, looking for answers to this question. Setting an intention or asking a positive-framed question, in the form of the brain wavelength called *delta*, where the conscious and subconscious mind interact, creates an intent the brain and body will work to create in reality.

3—Get in the Flow

A *flow state* is when a person is hyper-focused on satisfying a single task or activity. All their energy and attention are directed toward the task, and few thoughts about themselves or their performance offer any distraction. Athletes often refer to this as being "in the zone."

Psychologist Mihály Csíkszentmihályi published his research on flow in his book *Flow*. In a TED Talk, he has called it the "secret to happiness."[18] Flow is a state of optimal experience that can be integrated into our everyday lives. Flow is analogous with mindfulness; both help us focus attention and energy on the present moment during a task or activity. However, a person can be in a state of mindfulness regardless of whether they are completing a task.

We can find a state of flow while doing virtually any activity, whether it's gardening, needlework, walking, playing sports, reading a book, swinging on a swing, lying in the grass looking at the clouds, playing board games, or riding a bike. Flow states are not reserved for major events that require time to be set aside. They simply require the intent to be present and create a sense of purpose with the task at hand. I achieve a flow state when riding my horse, doing, yoga, swimming, and, oddly enough, sweeping the floor.

My older daughter gets into the zone when costume designing, and even running around appearing to be a scatter-brained teen. She is in her glory when she is doing what she loves, in her flow. Designing costumes is fast paced and intense, but she is focused and feels accomplished, which boosts her sense of wellness and healing. When she struggled with her condition and was unable to go to classes, her dad and I would let her go to theater because she could get into a flow state. Our decision paid off: Her socializing while creating a flow state, coupled with music and meditation, played a big role in her path to healing.

Flow can be found with anything that brings you a sense of purpose. I have found that using music helps me induce flow. While writing this book, I used music to create flow. Combining music and a flow task is my favorite approach.

4—Sleep as If Your Life Depends on It, Because It Does

Adequate amounts of restorative sleep are crucial to boosting our emotional, and physical, immune systems. The key word here is *restorative*. Restless or interrupted sleep doesn't do the trick. Our mind and body use deep sleep to restore connections in the brain, to send healing messages throughout the body, and to prepare our immune system for the next day. Therefore, sleep is critical to healing.

Unfortunately, our generation struggles with sleep, even considering all-nighters a badge of honor. All too often, we fall asleep with the television or other media playing intense material that keeps our stress system alert. New mothers (and fathers) are perfect examples. When they bring their infant home, for the first few months they struggle with obtaining restorative sleep, and their moods and physical wellness can suffer. One study demonstrated that sleep quality among college students predicted both positive and negative dimensions of mental health, with worse sleep being associated with higher levels of depression and lower well-being.[19]

Nowadays, we are more aware of contagions and how to protect ourselves: washing our hands after being in busy airports or touching public restroom door knobs, covering our mouths when coughing, and so on. But I hope I have convinced you that we need to give equal attention to boosting our emotional immune system as well. The health of our own mindset can positively affect the happiness of those around us.

Chapter Five

What Kind of Parent Are You?

Helicopter, Bulldozer, Avoidant, or Lighthouse?

Like most parents, Mary loved her daughter, June. But Mary translated her love into being overly protective, even though she believed she was just doing the right things. She went above and beyond the call of duty, kid-proofing the high chair; fencing off the stairs; locking drawers, closets, and doors; and rearranging all objects so they could not fall to the ground, lest June get hit in the head or step on broken ceramic. Every meal was carefully calculated with just the right amount of nutrients, and there was no room for sugary desserts. Mary also dressed June extremely safely, with no belts or clips or anything that could catch an edge and drop June to the floor or get caught in her hair. On top of this, Mary never let June out of her sight. No babysitter or extended family member was allowed to watch June without Mary's own supervision. Mary's fears prevented June from experiencing life outside of this bubble.

Can you imagine how Mary's treatment, a parenting attachment style called the *Helicopter*, could affect June? I get it—parents aren't perfect, and we all want what's best for our children. But can attachment go too far? What if it does not go far enough? And what are the repercussions of your parenting attachment style?

In this chapter, I discuss four parenting attachment styles so you can see where you may land. First, a little background: The term *attachment styles* refers to the way primary caregivers interact with their young children and how those interactions affect their well-being, and relationships, as they age. A *secure attachment* is a special emotional relationship that involves an exchange of comfort, care, and pleasure. John Bowlby devoted extensive research to secure attachments, describing them as a "lasting psychological connectedness between human beings."[1]

A 2012 study revealed that adolescents with the greatest empathic responsiveness had low levels of attachment insecurity and high levels of *vagal tone*.[2] Vagal tone is a physiologic index of emotion regulation. In other words, your attachment style as a parent influences your child's mental, emotional, and physical health. This study referred to the *vagus nerve*, the nerve that connects the brain to the gut, one that plays an important role in maintaining the body's homeostasis and influences cardiac function, as discussed in Chapter 1. There is a link between vagus nerve activity and heart rate variability (HRV) that correlates with vagal tone. What does this mean? HRV is simply a measure of the variation in time between each heartbeat. This variation is controlled by a primitive part of the central nervous system, the autonomic nervous system (ANS). Recall from Chapter 1 that the ANS is one of the four major players in the mind–body connection.

Vagal tone is a clinical measure that indicates overall levels of vagal nerve activity but is measured indirectly through HRV. Low vagal tone is indicative of an activation of the limbic system's fight, flight, or freeze response. High vagal tone is linked to the activation of the parasympathetic nervous system's rest-and-digest function (see Chapter 1).

What does any of this have to do with your parenting attachment style? Your style of parenting affects your child's HRV/vagal tone. Your parenting style can shake and vibrate the vagus nerve, changing the time between heartbeats, resulting in low HRV, poor vagal tone, and emotion dysregulation. This has a direct correlation to your child's health. Let's say your parental attachment style creates in your child a series of automatic negative thoughts (ANTs). These thoughts create emotions, and emotions create a cascade of hormones and chemical reactions that innervate every cell in the body. Your child can catch your vibes and repeated stressors; unhealthy parental attachment styles affect vagal tone, influencing the mind–body connection either positively or negatively. We know prolonged stress and emotion dysregulation are linked to both diseases and the disease process.

So, understanding, and perhaps modifying, your parenting attachment style is key to your child's health and development. There are four major types of attachment styles, and I've added colloquial terms to make them easier to identify.

- Bulldozer and Helicopter (anxious attachment)

- Avoidant (dismissive–avoidant attachment)

- Disorganized (fearful–avoidant attachment)

- Lighthouse (secure attachment)

Evidence strongly suggests that your attachment style is directly correlated with the type of childhood and parenting style that you had as a child. Also interesting is the fact that the attachment style you have with your romantic partner is the same attachment style you have with your children. For example, if you are avoidant with your partner, you are probably avoidant with your child.

Before we get to know these attachment styles, let me offer a word of caution. Please know my intent is to empower you to identify with, and change, any and all areas that may be negatively impacting your child and bring awareness to you and your family life so you and your child can heal! So, if you feel your blood pressure rising or start to become uncomfortable or even upset with me and want to defend your rights as a parent, that's normal. Even if you fear, deep down inside, that you may have work to do, be encouraged that change isn't always easy. But it can be extremely beneficial.

The Bulldozer Parent: A Form of Anxious Attachment

A Bulldozer parent is characterized by an anxious attachment style and seeks to remove all obstacles from a child's path so they don't experience pain, failure, or discomfort. These parents are overprotective and overly involved. The motivation behind Bulldozer parenting comes from a place of genuine deep love and concern. On the basis of my expertise and experience, a Bulldozer parenting style stems from the parent's subconscious fear of either failure and/or that their children's failure will be a direct reflection of them as parents. Parents who adopt this style believe that they are protecting and helping their children from hardships and setting them up for success (thereby making themselves look good, too). These well-intentioned parents aim to ensure a smooth, obstacle-free path for their children, intervening at the slightest sign of difficulty or distress. The increasing competitiveness in education, sports, the arts, college admissions, and the job market may contribute to this parenting approach, as parents try to do anything to get their children a leg up in this cutthroat modern-day culture of competitiveness.

As a mom whose children once attended an elite private school, I saw this every day and definitely felt the strong urge to try this attachment style to help my kids in a highly competitive, albeit dysfunctional, intense school environment. So, I hold zero judgment for this very common approach. In this elite private school, I witnessed over the years so many parents do their kids' homework, lie about audition times and locations to give their kid a leg up, line pockets, and pay for extra lessons in addition to the 3 hours day of practice for their 8-year-old.

The irony of the Bulldozer parent is that their style breeds, at exponential levels, anxiety, depression, low self-esteem, low self-efficacy, and autoimmune (AI) and functional gastrointestinal (GI) issues. All these issues were at epidemic levels in the private school and in upper middle-class communities where my children and I lived. That school served as a microcosm of what I see in the world and in my practice.

The largest percentage of patients I treat have Bulldozer parents. I'd estimate that more than 80% of my patients have at least one Bulldozing parent mixed with a Helicopter-type, "be careful" parenting style I discuss next.

Bulldozer parenting can have unintended consequences. By constantly clearing the path for their children, parents inadvertently hinder their child's ability to develop essential life skills, resilience, self-reliance and, most important, grit, my favorite personality trait that I love to see fostered in children. I have seen a Bulldozing parent overly involved in their child's social life, getting into teenage drama and theatrics and even calling other teenagers in a fit of rage, much to their child's utter embarrassment. Needless to say, that child's GI tract was a wreck afterward.

Bulldozing is an unhealthy form of codependency and enmeshment. *Enmeshment* is when boundaries between the parent and child are blurred. This results in a lack of autonomy and individual identity, which is critical for social, emotional, and psychological development. The child of a Bulldozer parent lacks the ability to to develop their own sense of self. I've treated the fallout from this type of parenting, from 16-year-olds who refuse to drive to 18- to 22-year-olds who refuse to go away to college—or, worse yet, have to return home because they can't make their way without their parents. The harsh reality of the real world becomes crushing, and their health tanks. That's when I get the call, and I have the honor of empowering the child to achieve self-efficacy. It is so rewarding to see a young human grow into themselves. I was once asked, "If I could give every child one gift, what would it be?" My reply: "The gift of failure."

In my own life, I have encouraged my kids to reach for something high, far from their reach but obtainable. It was extremely painful to see the tears and pain from them failing, but it built their grit and taught them how to stand back up again after the long fall. It taught them the knowledge that "It's OK not to be OK." I like to ask Bulldozer parents, "If someone cleared all your obstacles your entire life, would you be where you are in life and have the wisdom and knowledge you possess?"

The caveat to my discussion of Bulldozing is that I'm not suggesting that you ignore your child's safety. Parenting is not an easy role, so finding a healthy, reasonable balance will require a few more tears, and perhaps guidance from a mentor or counselor.

The Helicopter Parent: Another Form of Anxious Attachment

If you find yourself saying, "Be careful" a lot, you may fall into the Helicopter parenting style, which is a close cousin to the Bulldozer style and is also characterized by an anxious attachment style. While the Bulldozer parent clears a safe path and is overly protective of their child, removing all obstacles and tasks for the child, the Helicopter parent is overly involved as the child tries to complete the tasks or obstacle, hovering over them—well, like a helicopter. This includes being overly protective, insisting on strict supervision, always assessing risk, and making decisions for their children. In effect, Helicopter parents are hovering over every aspect of their children's life.

For example, the Helicopter parent will remind their child who is on a playground that meets all modern-day safety standards, "Be careful, Johnny;

don't fall!" When I hear this, I have to hold back with every fiber of my being from stating, "Your child inherently KNOWS not to fall. It's a natural instinct we were all born with." This style is repeated, over the course of the child's life, instilling and imposing fear where there was once childlike wonderment, exploration, fun, freedom, and a natural child-like curiosity and exploration. Overcoming simple fears, like swinging high on the swing set, is actually developmentally important, even if at the peak of the upswing you experience your stomach drop for a millisecond. I have asked many of my child patients if they have ever done this, or even know how to ride a bike with no hands, or pop a wheelie, and the number who say "No" breaks my heart.

A parent who creates an anxious attachment with their child often experienced this style of attachment themselves as a child. Their own emotional needs, which were not consistently met, left them feeling empty. So, they overcompensate by showering what they believe to be extra love and attention upon their children. They overcompensate to fill the emotional hole from their own childhood, which lacked love, attention, and safety.

Helicopter parenting sends resounding messages and automatic negative thoughts (ANTs) to your child, such as *I can't trust myself. My mom (or dad) doesn't trust me not to fail. There's no way I can trust myself if they don't trust me.* Children who grow up under these conditions lack the ability to make decisions; have high anxiety, a fear of failure, and a fear of making mistakes; and ultimately believe they are not good enough. Oftentimes, the Helicopter parenting style fosters phobias and obsessive-compulsive disorder, along with numerous ANTs.

When we repress fear and anxiety, we think, in essence, that they are stored away, but they are actually being dealt with internally, which fosters disease. Children grow up believing they can't trust their instincts or gut because their parents were involved with every decision and were told what to do and when and how to do it. The simple, caring phrase "Be careful" backfires, and so these children learn to ignore their gut, even their survival instincts. There is no independent thinking, autonomous choices, or outside free time or downtime (without devices) to explore, play, fall, get dirty, climb too high in a tree, or hang upside down from a swing set. All the things that cause a little natural fear in children, that build confidence, grit, and self-efficacy, are not allowed to come into fruition or be experienced. They doubt themselves. Their grades, friends, and achievements show that they are successful, but their symptoms tell a different story. They internally get sick with anxiety and worry, leading to irritable bowel syndrome (IBS), inflammatory bowel disease, constipation, and migraines.

A parental bond characterized by insecure attachment (Bulldozing or Helicopter) ironically fails to meet a child's need for safety, security, understanding, and calmness. It also robs them of having the chance to solve problems on their own and learn self-efficacy. The mindset of self-efficacy is "I'll figure it out." Low self-efficacy is directly related to higher levels of anxiety; people with high levels of self-efficacy have low levels of anxiety. Preventing a child's developing brain from organizing itself in the best ways, through overparenting, can inhibit emotional, mental, and even physical development, leading to difficulties in learning and forming healthy relationships later in life.

The majority of patients I've treated have found maladaptive ways to cope with insecure attachment styles, often by becoming overachievers. A deep core need is to seek relief from the pressure to prove they are good enough. They never feel good enough, no matter how much they do. They grow to believe that because their parents, Bulldozer or Helicopter, do everything for them, the parents believe the child is not capable, that the child can't get anything right, or do anything well enough. My patients regularly express that because their parents have done everything for them, they must be stupid, or incompetent. If parents don't trust their children, or don't empower their children to accomplish things and, more important, fail on their own or, worse yet, not meet the parents' expectations and standards, then how can these children trust themselves? These children develop maladaptive responses so they can please people; earn love and approval; and prove how good, smart, and capable they are.

Overbearing love creates a need for perfectionism to help recalibrate the attachment imbalance. These children internalize their fears and beliefs, and they work overtime to please their parents in an attempt to feel a sense of self-worth and gain parental favor. They use their fear of failure to create an internal dialogue that feeds the ANTs, ANTs that stir up a stress and limbic response. Then, an emergency relief valve is sought in the form of secondary gains by creating somatic symptoms of anxiety and illnesses. This grants them relief from their fears of failure, of the sense of not being good enough. It's like a "Get Out of Jail Free" card: *I'm too sick to go do what they want from me, to be perfect. I can't maintain perfection. I am not good enough to be perfect. If I'm sick, I don't have to do everything they expect of me.* These are the most common phrases I hear, from all ages, and the most common expressions of secondary gain. I will explore this more in a later Chapter 7.

Anxious attachment styles are formed in early childhood and have profound effects on a child's emotion regulation, stress responses, and overall health. An anxious attachment develops in children whose caregivers are overly anxious or nervous, leading to a heightened need for reassurance and closeness. As adults, they may exhibit clinginess, a fear of abandonment, and heightened emotional sensitivity. Here are some means by which the anxious attachment style affects an individual's mental and physical well-being:

- *Somatic symptoms.* The ongoing anxiety associated with this attachment style can manifest physically as headaches, stomachaches, muscle tension, or even heart palpitations. These symptoms are often exacerbated in stressful situations, particularly those involving relationships.

- *Heightened anxiety.* People with anxious attachment are more likely to experience generalized anxiety disorder and panic attacks because of their heightened emotional sensitivity and fear of rejection.

- *GI issues.* The chronic stress and anxiety associated with anxious attachment can disrupt digestive function, leading to conditions like IBS or other GI disorders.

- *Immune system suppression.* The prolonged activation of the stress response system can suppress the immune system, making a person more susceptible to infections and AI conditions.

The Avoidant Parent: Dismissive–Avoidant Attachment

Children who have an Avoidant parent, with a dismissive–avoidant attachment style, lack connection to them or caregivers and may be especially likely to be estranged from their parents in adulthood.[3] The Avoidant parent's style is characterized by distance, and they are largely out of tune with their children's needs. In turn, they cause their children considerable distress. Avoidant parents may give their child the silent treatment, avoid communication, or invalidate how the child feels. *Chronic invalidation* is a term used to describe a situation in which a person's emotions, thoughts, and experiences are repeatedly dismissed or ignored. A parent who tells their child that their emotions are wrong or they "shouldn't feel that way" is dismissing and invalidating the child's human experience. Chronic invalidation can lead to a range of mental health issues, and it can have physical consequences. Repeated invalidation can erode a person's sense of self-worth and cause them to doubt their own experiences. Over time, this can lead to chronic health issues.

Children learn to adapt to this style of feeling rejected and, in turn, they build defensive attachment strategies in an attempt to feel safe; to modulate or tone down intense emotional states; and to relieve anger, frustration, and pain. They often are estranged from their parents as adults, to relieve the pain from their childhood rejection. Their repressed pain, anger, sadness, caused by a lack of connection and chronic invalidation, creates a disruption in vagal tone and, over time, can be expressed as disease.

Children of Avoidant parents are by far the most painful to treat because the dismissive–avoidant attachment pattern leaves the child confused and enraged and feeling like they are the problem, that they are not worthy of love (thereby creating and exacerbating ANTs). Personally, at times, I feel a great empathy for both the child and the parent because the parent must be in great pain as well. They were probably raised this way themselves, and this typically pours over into the way they treat their partner. These parents avoid their child's emotions because of their own limited emotional capacity. They lack the capacity to handle their own emotions and have limited bandwidth to hold space for their child's needs unless the child is expressing happiness or gratitude. Avoidant parents may exhibit angry outbursts and emotion dysregulation disproportionate to the event. This drives people-pleasing behaviors in their children, who wish to avoid angering the parent, and creates immense anxiety in children, who wonder what they have done to deserve the silent treatment. This breeds and nourishes insecurities and the core belief that they are not good enough, not worthy, and not lovable, thereby creating immense stress.

Dismissive–avoidant attachment is one of the most damaging styles to the people whom love you the most. It often takes the form of withholding affection and communication with punitive intent. The silent treatment and emotion stonewalling has been shown to cause structural changes in the brain, which is brain damage, in other words.[4]

Avoidant parents will most often not hold themselves accountable for their actions, words, or behaviors and will blame others, their spouse, or their children for any discord, conflict, or break in the connection. They will let days go by without any meaningful contact between them and their children. Instances of loving, fun interactions are rare and often laced with disappointment for both parent and child. I see that children of Avoidants often have AI disorders, such as optic neuritis, because they have repressed anger toward the Avoidant parent. This is an exceptionally damaging parental style for children, who are forced to be exposed to emotional outbursts, stonewalling, the silent treatment, and a lack of accountability.

A case comes to mind of a patient of mine, a 16-year-old boy named Barry, who had an Avoidant father who would feel personally attacked when Barry expressed a need to spend more time with him or to receive better communication from him. Barry would ask for a simple call or text from the father, who was working late, to just check in, to hear his voice. His father worked long hours by choice, and Barry simply craved a real connection with him, but the father would become enraged when Barry would ask for more of his time. Barry would ask for time, and the father would vacillate in his responses, either becoming rageful or ignoring his request altogether, shaming Barry into silence. To avoid being an emotional burden to the man he loved and admired so much, Barry retreated into a world of hyper-independence. As soon as he was old enough, and no longer needed his father's financial support, he estranged himself from his father in order to protect his mental health and peace of mind. He learned to live without the lack of emotional safety and intimacy he so craved and deserved and had once begged for. He eventually stopped begging for his father's time and attention, and he now is in full recovery from his optic neuritis, living life as a successful attorney. The way an adult child treats their parents is often indicative of the treatment they received as a child; it's a mirrored reflection.

Avoidant parents love their children with all their hearts and would "do anything for them," advocate for them, solve problems, find solutions, and show immense amounts of love—at times. Avoidants love the way *they feel* others should be loved, not the way their children (or partner) *need* to be loved. There is love, lots of it, but the Avoidant just has a maladaptive way of showing it.

This is why the inconsistency is so confusing for children. A child will wait for bread crumbs of approval and connection, walking on eggshells trying to please the parent. An Avoidant parent simply lacks the bridge between mature accountability and emotional vulnerability. This isn't always intentional; it often is due to a lack of inner healing work and projections of their own traumas. They may be emotionally distant, struggle with intimacy, and prefer independence over closeness. Maybe you even experienced something like this growing up yourself?

In an effort to protect themselves from potential rejection, people with Avoidant parents may numb their emotions. This emotional numbness can extend to a reduced awareness of physical sensations, including pain, which can delay the recognition and treatment of health issues. Here are additional consequences of the Avoidant attachment style:

- *Internalized anxiety.* Although Avoidant individuals may appear calm on the surface, they often experience internalized anxiety, which can contribute to issues such as high blood pressure, cardiovascular problems, or chronic tension.

- *Chronic pain.* The suppression of emotions and stress can contribute to chronic pain conditions, particularly in the neck, shoulders, and back, as the body stores unprocessed emotions.

- *Weakened immune response.* Like those with anxious attachment, Avoidant individuals may experience a weakened immune response due to the chronic stress of emotional suppression, leading to increased susceptibility to infections and slower recovery times.

Both anxious and avoidant attachment styles can lead to long-term mental and physical health issues if not addressed. Chronic stress, whether due to hyper-arousal or emotion suppression, disrupts the body's natural healing processes, leading to a range of health problems, including anxiety disorders, chronic pain, GI issues, and immune system dysfunction.

If you feel that you or the other parent has an Avoidant parenting style, that's OK, because it's OK not to be OK. There is always time to heal your own wounds in order to help your child heal from theirs. All we can ask of ourselves as parents is we strive to be better no matter what style we operate from. I made a promise to my children at a very young age after I had made an epic parental mistake: "I promise you one thing in life, I promise I will make a million more mistakes, but I also promise I will not repeat them."

The Disorganized Parent: Fearful–Avoidant Attachment

The Disorganized parent is characterized by a fearful–avoidant attachment style that often develops in children who experience inconsistent, frightening, or emotionally neglectful caregiving. The Disorganized parent can vacillate between kind and loving to yelling the next moment. I see this in about two out of every 10 patients. These parents love their children dearly and have no idea that they are operating from this form of attachment style. If I were to venture a guess, I would say that if these parents had the awareness, they would be devastated and ashamed. Disorganized parents often seem very attentive and loving in public, but behind closed doors their children experience the aspects of the parent no one else sees. These children may oscillate between seeking closeness and withdrawing, often feeling confused or fearful in relationships with their caregivers. Children raised by Disorganized parents can experience significant disruptions in connections to their caregiver (or parents). Early experiences of fear, confusion, or neglect can lead to chronic activation of a complex stress response system, which affects both psychological and physical health. Parents characterized by anxious, avoidant, and disorganized attachment styles may notice the following repercussions in their children:

- *Stress response.* Children raised by people whose parenting is characterized by disorganized attachment are often in a state of heightened alertness; their nervous system is constantly scanning for threats (neuroception) because of past experiences with unpredictable caregiving. This chronic stress can lead to an overactive sympathetic nervous system, which may result in ongoing anxiety, difficulty relaxing, and poor sleep—all of which negatively affect health.

- *GI disorders.* Chronic stress can disrupt the digestive system, leading to conditions such as IBS or other GI issues.

- *AI diseases.* The constant stress and lack of emotional support can weaken the immune system, making the body more susceptible to AI diseases.

- *Chronic pain.* The fearful–avoidant attachment that characterizes Disorganized parents has been linked to the development of chronic pain conditions, whereby unresolved emotional distress and anxiety manifest as physical pain, particularly in the muscles and fascia.[5]

Children raised by Disorganized parents often struggle with severe anxiety. Their early experiences teach them that the world is unpredictable and that they cannot reliably depend on others for comfort or safety. As they grow older, this internalized sense of insecurity can evolve into generalized anxiety, social anxiety, or even panic disorders. Disorganized parenting is also associated with difficulties in managing emotions. These children may have intense emotional reactions to stress, and they may struggle to calm themselves, further exacerbating anxiety. The unresolved emotional distress associated with Disorganized parenting and the fearful–avoidant attachment on which is is based can manifest physically.

Without intervention, the impacts of Disorganized parenting can persist into adulthood, leading to difficulties in forming healthy relationships, maintaining mental health, and managing physical health. Adults with a fearful–avoidant attachment style may also be at higher risk for developing severe mental health issues, such as depression, post-traumatic stress disorder, and borderline personality disorder.[6]

If you feel you may be a Disorganized parent, it is OK. Many loving parents have a fearful–avoidant type of attachment style; this does not negate your love for and commitment to your child. It simply may illustrate you had a Disorganized parent growing up, and this is your survival mechanism as well. Awareness with no judgment is the key to unlocking the tools that may help your child heal.

The Lighthouse Parent: Secure Attachment

The Lighthouse parent is a stable, consistent beacon of light, looking out across the shoreline as their children navigate the waters of life. They have invested in their children and prepared them to ride the waves of life, but they shine a light on the dangers so their children do not crash against the rocks. They have invested in themselves and trust their abilities as a parent. They trust their children (as appropriate for their children's age) to make the right choices, and when a child inevitably makes poor choices they have enough bandwidth, time, and calm energy to be present for them and guide them through the rough storm. Lighthouse parents strike a balance among loving their children, protecting them, communicating with them, nurturing healthy boundaries, and giving them the confidence and freedom to navigate parts of the storm on their own. This fosters and builds in their children self-reliance, trust, self-efficacy, and a secure sense of autonomy. A Lighthouse parent is a stable, strong, and reliable source of guidance. They don't take the helm, or resort to saying "Be careful," and they don't try to make the storm or rocky shores disappear; they simply guide their children and help them navigate their way to safety. A Lighthouse parent will say, "Be mindful of the consequences. I trust you to make the right choice, and trust yourself. You've got this, and I'm here if you need me." Or, they will ask this question, which puts children in a position to be mindful of their needs: "What can I do for you at this moment?"

The Lighthouse parent has done the hard work of self-awareness with a commitment to self-growth, developing and evolving as humans and as parents. They put the work into their own mental health, their wounds, and other traumas, and they practice self-care of mind, body, and spirit. They serve as a model, as a beacon of light for the child. They prioritize their own mental health and are mentally resilient to not catching other's vibes. They may have failed many times, and they are OK with not being OK. They can openly admit their failures and fears, and take accountability for their actions, behaviors, and flaws. They are safe in their own skin, and their children feel emotionally safe in their presence.

A secure attachment bond ensures that your children will feel safe, understood, and calm enough to experience the optimal development of their nervous system. They feel a sense of safety that results in an eagerness to learn; a healthy self-awareness; trust; empathy; high self-efficacy and confidence; and good mental, emotional, and physical health.

As you can imagine, the Lighthouse parenting style benefits both the parents and their children and is the style to which parents ought to aspire.

Chapter Six

Back In "My Generation"

The Global Rise in Stress, Pressure, and Cyberpsychology

The most common theme I hear from overwhelmed, desperate parents is "Why is this happening to my child!?!" Well, the truth is no one can, with concrete evidence, point to one factor. Disease involves a combination of possibilities. Then the next stream of thoughts goes like this: "Well, back in my day, no one had allergies, autoimmune diseases, GI [gastrointestinal] issues, or talked about emotions. We all just got along, or we fought it out, and came home when the street lights came on."

My reply is always, "I agree; those were simpler times. Also, there is no way we can understand the immense amount of fears, pressure, and stress children are under, ranging from modern-day domestic national threats to their neighborhood schoolyard active-shooter threats as well as performance, sports, dance, and music school expectations; social media influences; and pressure starting in third grade to get into a good college. We actually have no comprehension of modern threats, pressures, and expectations."

Understandably, this is when the parents, sometimes the dad in particular, feel upset. Their child has a loving home, food, clothes, and most likely anything the child could possibly dream of: toys, bikes, devices, vacations, sports, dance lessons, and so on. I tell parents that I agree: There is no denying their child is well-cared for, so very loved, and that all their physical needs are met. That still does not negate their fears, pressures, expectations, stress, and the automatic negative thoughts (ANTs) that run unbridled in their minds. Both truths can exist on the same plain.

The next stream-of-consciousness thought I often hear expressed is "My child should be more grateful for ALL they have." I am the first to agree with this one, and yes, your children can still be grateful for all you provide. But we cannot discount that they are growing up in different times, times that breed fears, stress, pressures, expectations, and ANTs. Remember how I mentioned in Chapter 1 that a baby will coo at a caregiver but cry at a stranger? The baby shouldn't feel fear but does. We don't tell an infant they shouldn't feel fear; instead, we comfort them.

Being grateful helps, yes, but it won't negate the fears and ANTs that are the driving forces in your child's life. (Yet, by the end of this book, and after some practice, you and your child likely will marinate in gratitude for this healing journey rather than enduring fears of the unknown.)

So, with all that is provided to them, why are children still stressed or struggling with anxiety or depression?

Imagine back to what your kindergarten year felt like. Really stop and feel, smell, and recall. . . What did kindergarten *feel* like for you? The smell of the bottled glue, crayons, smashed PB-and-J sandwiches, tin lunch boxes with a plastic Thermos, extra-long recess times, and maybe even nap time? Do you remember what you learned in kindergarten? I don't—not much, really. I recall getting my "b"s and "d"s backward and being upset about not making the "clean plate club" and not getting my name recognized at lunch for it. Beyond that, there is not much I can recall. I have no clue what reading level I was at, or even what age I was when I began reading.

Now, fast forward to the post–9/11 era. Imagine—really stop and imagine, from a 5-year-old's perspective. Each year, our schools, media, churches, synagogues, and mosques recognize and honor the single worst event to happen in our country's history. These highly impressionable minds are exposed to images of actual planes hitting iconic buildings, flames, humans jumping out of buildings, and they just now are realizing that *this* is the world they are growing up in. I am NOT making a political or educational stance; I am highlighting the limbic part of the brain that is responsible for alerting us to danger and becoming engaged in this at such an early and unnecessary age. Society as a whole exposes and teaches our kids, year after year, that the world is full of terrorists and other humans who want to kill them. To the child's mind, they consciously and subconsciously register that the world is not safe. In short, our children are growing up believing the world is a threat.

Now, let's focus on closer, national threats in our hometowns. Kindergarten-age children go to school and are trained at age 5, and sometimes even younger, how to survive and hide if another human is shooting at them and trying to kill them and their friends. This all happens in between recess and nap time. Think about this—better yet, feel this as your child would. We send our children to school, and they practice, a few times a year, what to do if a person is attempting to mass-murder them and their friends. Now, go back again and recall and feel your kindergarten year. Does it feel the same? Please, really take a moment to imagine. Now, do that a few times a year over the course of 12 years, throwing in an actual active-shooter drill or threat a few times per year. As a child, you may have wondered if your sandwich was mushy by lunchtime, but your child is wondering *if someone is trying to kill me today.* These are real fears in the real world for our children that play a significant role in brain development. Again, I have zero interest in judging our nation, or our nation's school system. I am pointing out, from a neurobiological perspective, a contributing factor that is often overlooked in our child's socioemotional development that feeds into anxiety, depression, and, ultimately, autoimmune (AI) and GI diseases.

Our children see national and personal threats in the world, and now even their school is not safe. Even if your child is homeschooled, they are exposed to the knowledge of these threats and understand that kids their age are at risk. If your child is like almost all of my patients, they are most probably highly empathic. They feel safer at home, but they know kids their age are at risk for mass shootings. Children with AI and functional GI disorders are almost always highly empathic and can feel these secondary, or vicarious, fears. Just reading about this concept may contribute to a feeling of discomfort, setting off stress alarms in the mind and body. Now, multiply that feeling, because our children deal with this new reality every day.

Let's narrow the scope and laser in on the home environment. Imagine your child climbing the jungle gym or another apparatus in your backyard. With every grip and step, they are building psychomotor skills and self efficacy, which are critical skills. And, you just can't help yourself: You see them climb higher and higher. The tension builds. They are just about to take that first hard-to-reach leap of faith to grab that first bar. What is your instinctive inclination? While watching out the window with your coffee cup clenched tightly, you prepare to sprint into action wondering, *Is it time to remind little Johnny "Be careful!"?*

Or imagine this scenario. Your little Johnny is riding his bike on the sidewalk with a military-grade helmet on, of course (I had them for my kids, too) as he takes off to pedal as fast as his little legs can, gaining speed with freedom, excited yet with some trepidation, increasing speed every second. Think fast—what do you want to say? "Be careful Johnny! Not too fast!"

Now you are at the beach, and little Johnny runs to ankle-deep water to splash around and begins to get lost in the moment of joyful childhood play, but you are worried about sharks, stingrays, jellyfish, fish, and the undertow. What do you say to little Johnny? "Be careful, Johnny!" These examples highlight the anxious attachment style, which characterizes the "be careful" parent, also called a Bulldozer or Helicopter parent, discussed in Chapter 5.

So, our children have been taught that the world and our nation are not safe, school is not safe, and playing is not safe. They hear "Be careful" over and over through the years, with daily subconscious messaging. They can only ask themselves, *Is it safe to play now?*

Most children inherently know, from birth, that they do not want to fall from the monkey bars or be launched off their bikes. We are lovingly, unknowingly instilling fear where there once was childlike curiosity and chances to explore childhood and all the skinned knees and falls that come with the territory. Despite our best intentions to provide a safe environment and experience as our children explore the world, we are sending them a message: "I don't trust you, as you play, to not avoid the most basic, primal human instinct, to avoid pain."

The most natural thing a child can do is play, but these days we've ingrained into their mindset the notion that playing is dangerous. They lose trust in themselves; how can they trust themselves if you don't trust them? Free play, unstructured outdoor playtime, and imagination play is a way of life, long forgotten, and it is so critical to healthy brain development, self-efficacy, autonomy, and grit, as well as a key factor of intelligence called *adaptability*. Grit and adaptability are two major elements I see lacking in children of Bulldozer and Helicopter parents. They are fed a lifetime of fears, and those fears feed the

ANTs that nourish the stress-and-disease process. They will fall, they will fail, and most of the time they are OK in the end.

I am not suggesting a 1970s–1980s feral child upbringing. Instead, I suggest replacing "Be careful," with "Hey! Be mindful. You got this!" This difference builds awareness, self-reliance, an innate trust in the self, and confidence, and it shows your children that you trust them. The "Be mindful" phrase empowers your child and builds them up rather than creating a "Be careful" lifelong fear-based mindset.

Taking a broader approach to "back in my generation," most likely your parents watched the nightly news as dinner was being prepared. So, you had one hour a day of the world's problems per day. Contrast that with modern-day news, which is on 24/7. When my children were in sixth grade, the school even downloaded the news into the school-issued iPad to take home with them. They were pushed into having real-time access to the world's dark side as news stories broke and popped up on their screens while they were doing homework.

So, I instituted one major rule in my house: No exposure to the news. I told them I would inform them of major events, and we discuss them as a family. I know the neuroscience; the impact of stress contagion; and the influence of negative news on the brain, mind, and nervous system. It creates unnecessary fears and worries as children realize they have no control.

In my practice, children who are exposed to secondhand or firsthand news have higher anxiety scores. They self-report fears of becoming an adult, and when I see 19- to 22-year-olds with functional GI issues I have noted that they often have an inability to sustain adulting behaviors and a healthy, adaptive form of independence from their parents. They are often too scared of adulting, too scared to drive, and scared of the world in general. This creates a secondary gain whereby our youth avoid real-world responsibilities. They suspend the dangerous world of adulthood because they feel ill equipped to handle it, just as they couldn't—or were not permitted to—navigate childhood safety. So, their minds and bodies believe they aren't safe to be an adult. Being a kid wasn't safe, so how can adulting be? This fear of becoming an adult creates fears and stressors that the body mirrors inside the GI tract. If you have managed to filter the news with your child and provided healthy, dynamic conversations about real risks, keep up the good work! But make sure your face doesn't tell a different story. Research on emotion contagion has revealed that even our facial expressions can induce a change in the onlooker's emotional condition. These emotional conditions arise unconsciously, initiated by cues in the environment that distinctively affect people's mood.[1] Perhaps the most sinister of contagions comes from social media, where facial expressions, videos, memes, and vicious attacks illustrate the angst that exists in the world.

Back in my generation, we didn't have to contend with social media. But today's kids have 24/7 access to a wide range of "influencers" who specialize in stoking fears, sharing critical opinions, and shaming others. Unfortunately, negative messaging is far more popular than positive messaging. Our minds tend to veer toward negativity, even when we don't want to. I applaud parents who monitor their children's social media intake, at least until eighth or ninth grade. Those parents are protecting their children's mental health and potential disease consequences.

Our modern era has brought a new field of study: cyberpsychology. According to research conducted by J. R. Anics (2000), five major areas have been identified as being relevant to the field of cyberpsychology, including trends and directions in cyberpsychology ethics, research, training, and application.[2] These include:

1. Online behavior and personality

2. Social media use and psychological functioning

3. Games and gaming

4. Telepsychology

5. Virtual reality, artificial intelligence, and other applications.

Studies have shown that schoolchildren with increased time spent on either smartphones, social media, or gaming had significantly elevated psychological distress and anxiety symptoms.[3] As we know, anxiety and psychological distress are significantly related to exacerbation of AI and GI symptoms. My biggest fear as a mind–body therapist is when I see "sticky iPad kids," or toddlers, even babies, on a device at dinner or while sitting on their parent's lap. It simply breaks my heart knowing that that child is at a high risk for depression, anxiety, obesity, addiction, poor social connectedness, and diminished overall well-being. As our world becomes increasingly digitized, the field of cyberpsychology has been growing. We do know that limiting social media and device use is beneficial in reducing the risk of depression, anxiety, and mental distress.

Grades and competition could be an entire book of its own. My oldest had mysterious GI and bladder issues that started (and ended) in third grade when grading of the students' schoolwork began. All she wanted was to get straight As, compete with her friends, and, more important, make us, her parents, happy. This was in 2015, before I began to work with GI patients. We ran all over town, to so many doctors, and even ended up in a neurology office, and this is when I got schooled. To be very transparent with my own parenting flaws, I was one of those moms, who in secret, kinda hidden, in a soft way, pressured my child to compete and have good grades even if I argued otherwise back then. I would ask, "How did you do on your test? Did you get an A?" With the benefit of hindsight, I know this added pressure to perform.

So, when we went to the neurology office, I told the doctor about her major milestones, family history, and what a great, easy kid she is—no behavioral issues, plays sports, has all As, and volunteers, too! Oh, and "she wants to go to Harvard and become a judge," I said boastfully. (If you remember from the previous chapter, she is a reflection of what a great parent I am.) The room became dead silent, and the doctor glared at me as his face got redder and redder. He was trying to control an outburst, and I saw it coming. He cleared his throat and, with an enraged expression, took a long pause and asked, "Why is your 8-year-old talking about college, let alone Harvard!?" Then he raised his voice: "I have a floor full of children her age with neurological problems just from stress! Do you want your kid in my hospital, too? DO you? If you keep this up, she'll be there soon. She shouldn't have a care in the world, she should be playing outside, not caring about her grades, lots of free down time, and no talk of college 'til high school!"

I was properly humbled, utterly embarrassed, and then, eventually, grateful. He was right, and I knew it. I took the beating with my chin up, eager to learn from him. I would do anything to help my child. I was making some epic mistakes as a mom and, 100 pediatric patients later, oh, boy, was I. We did a 180-degree turn from expectations and pressures and stopped all the college talk.

I removed her from some of her extracurricular activities, and freed up Saturdays and Sundays so my kids could be kids. The result was that they climbed trees more often, had picnics by the lake, played in the treehouse, hung out with the horses, rode bikes, built forts, ran barefoot, flew kites, and got dirty on the weekends. Like magic, her GI issues cleared up. They have never returned since.

I made a mental note of what not to do with my younger daughter, who was 6 years old at the time. For example, I have not checked my children's grades since that third-grade year. I literally do not even know how to access their grades. They are so proud of their hard work, and they show me their grades on a regular basis. But I don't ask to see them. Instead, I ask "How did you feel about your test?" or "How did it go?", and "I do expect you to be prepared for class." After fifth grade, they learned to navigate school, and I became their support staff. I won't be *that* parent again, boasting how great my kids are. I will state that their GPAs are noteworthy but that neither their dad nor I had anything to do with that. Their dad and I worked to instill confidence in them, to let them know that they can do anything if they want, and we gave them the space to fail. We supported them when they fell, held them during meltdowns, provided tutoring when needed, and reinforced the mindset that they are highly capable and that a healthy, balanced life is 'way more important than any GPA.

I had to admit how wrong I was to secretly pressure my children to keep up with outside pressures and expectations and the need to please me. When they can't wait to share their grades, I praise them for all their hard work and tell them that their grades are a testament to how hard work pays off. My over parenting about grades, getting a lead role in the school play, practicing harder with swimming, was hurting them, and I needed to change to help my children get better.

I have seen versions of my old parenting style in so many parents, and with great compassion I understand. It is always a challenging conversation to tell them, "So, your kids are super stressed about how much pressure you are un-intentionally putting on them, and their mental and physical health is deterio-rating. They are terrified to tell you because they think you will get defensive, invalidate them or, worse yet, that they will displease you. It's humbling to realize that having self-reflection as a parent is paramount, that the modern-day pressure of grades was nothing like it was back in my generation. Our parents didn't have minute-by-minute updates on late assignments or play-by-play test and quiz scores. Could you imagine your mom emailing you at school or texting you, 'Hey, why did you get an 82 on the spelling quiz; we studied all night'"?

As parents, we need to strive to find balance in supporting our children, instead of smothering them, while teaching them that accountability and hard work pay off. Back in my day, grades weren't that important until high school and, yep, we didn't have epidemic levels of AI and GI issues.

Here are some good phrases to help mentally disarm stress while supporting your child:

- "It's not your job to please me or make me happy with your grades."

- "I am more interested in your hard work and effort."

- "I am proud of your dedication to school but, more important, you should be proud of yourself."

How cool would it have been to hear those words when you were a child back in your day?

Chapter Seven

Top 10 Things Kids Wish You Knew

UNDERSTANDING SECONDARY GAINS AND WHY THEY MATTER

D o you *believe* you can heal? Do you *want* to heal?

I ask each of my patients these two, seemingly obvious, questions after we have established a sense of being teammates on the same journey, with me as their guide, and when they feel a safe and solid bond, enough to be vulnerable. I can tell by their answer where they are on the journey to wellness or if they will double-down on the path to disease. I also expose what automatic negative thoughts (ANTs) are presented, when we do a deeper exploration of what their authentic reply is.

Most people would think the answer would be, "Yes, of course! Yes, I WANT to heal!" But when I ask, I am not looking for a candid, quick reply. I am seeking the depths of their truths, with no judgment. I understand their darkest secrets deserve to be honored and revealed in a safe space so that those dark thoughts are freed from the shadows into the light. I have had these dark secret thoughts myself, and I know the power of the mind and the role it plays in disease. I see it all day at work and in my own children. There is no hiding when I know there is dark truth to the hidden gains of autoimmune (AI) and gastrointestinal (GI) conditions. More often than not, one of the secrets, which they may not even be able to verbalize, is that they actually prefer being sick.

You may be thinking, "NO way—what does my child gain from this condition? This is suffering, and my child is crying for help!" I completely agree with you. You are right. Your child is suffering and may be begging for relief. Both can be true and still coexist. The mind is dynamic and complex, and we have no X-rays to examine the subconscious mind, which holds so much power. We are just beginning to understand its abilities. So, your truth about your child can still be true; physical conditions and secondary gains can coexist simultaneously.

A *secondary gain* is defined as the advantage that occurs in addition to the real illness.[1] It is a psychological term that refers to a motivating factor influencing a patient in reporting symptoms or complaints of pain. To understand secondary gains, you need to understand human motivation. According to Abraham Maslow's Hierarchy of Needs,[2] human beings are motivated by three basic needs: safety/security, belongingness, and self-esteem.

- *Security* means avoiding (emotional and physical) harm and injury.

- *Belongingness* means being accepted and appreciated.

- *Self-esteem* and *self-efficacy* are about having positive feelings toward oneself.

Please note that these motivators do not require or include any type of conscious thinking on the part of the patient. Types of secondary gain include using illness for personal or emotional advantage; to receive nurturing; to meet emotional needs or obtain sympathy; to avoid responsibilities or perceived pressures; to maintain dysfunctional attachment styles (as we discussed in Chapter 5), or even to identify with, and relate to, a sick parent or a loved one.

By the time a child feels comfortable working with me to dig deeper than the obvious answer to "Do you want to heal?", they know I won't play the "inauthentic" game for too long. The space we create as a team is a place to learn, grow, heal, and face all parts of the subconscious mind that can help them heal. If a long pause ensues, I know they are running thoughts of self-doubt through their head and imagining what life would look like if they were healed as well as the increased expectations that would be placed upon them. Once we break down the facade of expected, standard answers we begin to unpeel the very complex mind, like a huge onion. It's this cathartic moment of relief and freedom when the child admits, out loud, their hidden truths. This may take some deep self-reflection and awareness. But all my clients who have healed from these lessons know when they uncover their secondary gains, it becomes a catalyst for changing their life.

I have had several patients who, once they became aware of their secondary gains, began to feel better and not tell their parents they feel better. This occurs for a few reasons: They are not ready to face the possible backlash caused by the knowledge that they could have been healed all this time, or they are not ready to reintegrate themselves into reality.

Recall my first patient, Ruthie, from Chapter 2: She was healed almost instantly. Although her parents were overjoyed, they were also confused, and slightly upset with her, when they incorrectly concluded that Ruthie's illness had been all "in her head" and that she had unnecessarily kept up the ruse of being sick. Actually, it's common for parents to think all that suffering could have been "easily" prevented. Well, no; that is not at all how the subconscious mind works. I have seen some patients get yelled at by their parents for getting better so quickly, who feel they are being lied to about the sickness being "made up." Then, the child withdraws and puts another wall up between them and the parents. We parents spend so much time on secure parental bonding techniques, yet these pediatric patients are too fearful to trust their parents with such dark, intimate knowledge. Children will keep their hidden lives from parents as they slowly adjust to their new, non-sick, life.

Secondary gains provide undiscovered guides to help us get unstuck. **They're an invitation to understand the advantages we receive from retaining problems instead of solving them.** Among the hundreds of possible secondary gains experienced by being sick, these are some of the more common:

- They get extra sleep.

- They get extra loving attention.

- They are able to avoid adulthood responsibilities.

- They get a reprieve from internal pressures to perform or please others.

- They receive extra time to complete homework or tests.

- People are friendlier, and more caring.

- Less is expected from them.

- Others, like friends and family, make extra efforts to spend time with them.

- Being sick allows them to avoid social situations, work, or anything they don't want to do.

- They can stay home and do less.

The most common secondary gain I see is that sickness eliminates the anxiety and stress caused by a fear of failure. By being sick, a child with an AI or GI condition does not have to worry about failure because they don't have anything to fail at.

To be clear, these children DO have a physical illness which, in many cases, has a correlation with chronic stress—whether internal or external. The secondary gains are the only "bonus" they receive. So, please do not expect your child to openly confess their secondary gains. They assume you will accuse them of faking the illness to get something in return. Then, they will get even sicker to prove to you it's not in their head, so it would be a mistake to suggest they are benefiting.

Trust me on this. I see it all day long. Children admit to me they are proving to their parents how sick they are so that they feel heard and seen. I can relate. I used to put black eyeliner under my eyes so I would look as sick as I felt. I thought no one could see my disease, and see I am sick, and I kept hearing how great I looked, but I was suffering inside. I longed to be understood—to even receive some level of sympathy from others.

Never underestimate the desire to feel validated and seen. Instead of "torturing" (a word choice I often hear) your child for a confession, you can ask, "Are there any needs you have that you feel I am not meeting?" or "With no judgment or consequences, what would you miss most about being sick? Time home with me, fear of driving, or going back to school full time, or back to lots of pressure?"

The takeaway point is that your child has hidden secondary gains to their illness, and creating a safe space for them to start opening up to you is a good start. Then you can gently navigate your way around the purpose of their secondary gains. I can't emphasize this enough: If you accuse your child, saying it's "all in their head" or that they are faking any of their symptoms, they will get sicker. I have seen children take themselves to the point of near death through GI issues that morphed into eating disorders. It's terrifying to witness. They spend their time in treatment centers or hospitals just to prove to their parents how sick they are.

When one of my patients resists sharing any secondary gains, I am absolutely OK with revisiting the issue with compassion later on. Most who say they are not ready to explore this yet will admit openly they are not ready to give up being sick and what need of theirs is met from being sick. They realize they can still "keep their illness" for as long as they like. This ironic twist is SO POWERFUL in helping them feel in control of the disease. If they have addressed and brought awareness to their hidden core, unmet needs, they can begin to starve the ANTs. They begin to feel in control, empowering themselves that they have choices—even if the choice is to be sick. They don't feel helpless and betrayed by their own bodies, and eventually they slowly begin to feel better because they have discovered their authenticity.

Authenticity is the bridge to self-awareness that connects us to our higher selves, to inner Divinity within all of us that enables us to heal. I will address in Chapter 11 why people choose to stay in the Victim role or phase of the disease process. When humans have problems and benefit from them, keeping the status quo seems easier than overcoming the issues.

There are more specific things your child wishes you, their parent, knew, but they may never tell you. In a therapy setting, I am bound by the laws of confidentiality not to reveal what my patients say unless they are being harmed or harming themselves. Still, I've summarized the answers I've received from the hundreds of patients I've worked with. Although they want open communication, they are scared of making matters worse and upsetting you, displeasing you, hurting your feelings, or disappointing you. In a therapy setting, however, I have the liberty of asking directly, "What do you wish your parents knew that would help you feel better?"

After reassuring them that I cannot tell their parents, the dam opens. Over the past 20 years I've started to hear the Top 10 most common answers, which I share below. Please read this list with an open heart and compassion, knowing your child is suffering. The odds are they feel at least one or more of these things and will not tell you.

To be transparent, I'm in the same boat as you. I ask my kids, every few months, "Is there anything I am doing you wish I could do better?" Plus, there are times when we need to bring in a third-party expert/therapist who understands the mind–body connection to illness.

While writing this book, just last night, my daughter replied, "Yes. I need your undivided attention. It's annoying me that you are always on your phone lately."

Well, she was right. I could list all the million reasons why I do not always give her my undivided attention and give an explanation for how my work pays for our lives. Instead, I check my ego at the door and make a mental note to carve out focused time to spend just with her—even if that means I must stay up later to get work done. After all, time with our children is precious. We only have 18 summers until they leave the nest, so I accept the truth and my flaws. I am indeed always on my phone or computer lately. That is the truth no matter the reason, or how justified it is. It's also my daughter's truth that she needs my attention. She wants to know and *feel* I care about her life and what she has to say. Her words are important to me. So, when I mention these Top 10 things kids wish you knew, please know, I am with you.

The Top 10 Things Every Child Wishes Their Parents Knew

1. **You stress me out, bad.** You are so worried all the time or have anxiety—or someone in my family is angry a lot. Most of the time I am happy and doing OK, then you get all stressed, no matter what it is about. It affects me, and I take on ALL your worries and stress and take them as my own. When you worry or get anxious, I feel your energy; I don't know how not to. You stress out so much, it makes me think that I must be stressed and worry, too. If my role model stresses, then I must, too. Model for me that you got this. You are balanced, and I am safe. I don't feel safe when you are anxious, worried, or stressed. The vibes I'm exposed to really affect my well-being. HELP ME by modeling gratitude instead of stress.

2. **I am a human being, not a human DOING.** Please take the hidden and implied overachieving life pressures off me. Please model for me that doing nothing is OK. Being "unbusy" is OK and does not mean I am a failure or that I am lazy. Please realize that all the pressure I am silently feeling to please you is hurting me. Even if you tell me it's OK, I still hold it all in. With everything I do, and being pressured for good grades, to fit in, to please everyone, I am silently suffering under the pressure and activities (even the ones I love to do so much). Please understand; please give me permission to feel like I can rest, or even fail.

3. **Show me how to not take everything personally.** When you're upset at life, like all the medical bills piling up, I need to know that I am not a burden for you. I know I add stress to your life for being sick, and I feel SO much guilt for being a burden to you. I need to hear, "It's not your job to make me happy, or feel responsible for our emotions as your parents." I want to hear, "You are a kid. Go be a kid. I got this." And, "You are safe. I got you. I will handle this." (I tell my kiddo now, "The bills and these expenses are "nonyurbusiness," aka none of your business.)

4. **Validate me, listen to me without fixing it, please.** You tell me I shouldn't feel a certain way and give me all the reasons why, along with your solutions, but it makes me feel like I am wrong, and that I can't trust myself or my emotions. Or I am not good enough to work through the emotion myself. I feel like I am stupid for feeling that way, and if I can't trust my own feelings, what can I trust? I now feel like a failure to you, when you tell me why my feelings shouldn't be that way. Model for me that not being OK is OK. Show me that it's OK to feel emotional pain or discomfort and how to move that through me so it doesn't get stuck in me. Please let me be scared. I don't want to have to have to be strong or brave all the time. That is SO much pressure that I feel like I am letting you down again.

5. **I need guidance on discovering who I AM.** This includes *my*

interests, not what everyone else thinks or expects of me. Expectations keep me up and night and haunt me daily. Teach me how to rely on myself and grow my independence separate from you. I am so attached to you but, secretly, I want to be free at some level. I have no idea how to become me and not disappoint YOU. That fear terrifies me. I feel like if I pull away from you, become me, I will be lost, and you will be mad at me.

6. **I wish our home was my sanctuary.** I wish we spent more time connecting as a family, not just running around together. When we do connect over dinner, it becomes all about how I could be doing better, or why am I not eating enough, or what I can do to feel better. It's always about something I need to improve on: my grades, my homework, or a life lesson. I wish we could laugh, play games, and connect as people who like each other. Instead of rushing from place to place, can we just be at home, laugh, talk, without all the life lessons, stressful conversations, and unspoken tension over something? I wish we could just be a family once a week (or more) to just connect, without discussing all the bad news in the world and around us. During these times, I don't want anybody else with us, no additional relatives or friends. And I don't want to hear anyone complain about their life, bills, and work. No arguing! I just want to hang out with you like you would with an old friend, and enjoy my company—who I am as a person. Model for me what relaxed, safe fun looks like.

7. **I DO NOT want to have to be strong or brave.** I feel so much pressure to be brave and strong as I go through more tests. I don't want to be placed in a position to disappoint you. Realize that if I feel scared, alone, or trapped in my body that is betraying me that no one understands, I feel like no one understands me. If I am not brave or strong, that puts pressure on you because you worry about me, and I don't want to worry you more. So I carry the burden pretending I am strong and cry alone in my room or shower. I wish you knew how scared I am, how alone I feel, how helpless I am. Stop telling me I shouldn't be. I just am, and that is OK.

8. **Be real, and authentic, with me.** Being fake, pretending to smile when you are in emotional pain, is frustrating. I can tell when you are being fake to me or to people out in the world. When you act fake, it makes me feel like I have to be fake, too, in order to please you.

9. **Please stop telling other people about my illness.** It seems dramatic, and it embarrasses me. I feel like you do it for attention, telling others how hard it is on you, on me, and on the family. It just makes me feel worse, and more like a burden. And please stop posting about my illness and related updates. (Note: Oversharing and talking about your child's illness can be a form of secondary gain for the parent, to gain sympathy for all they have gone through with the AI or GI diagnosis. Ask your child's permission to tell *their* story.)

10. **Stop saying, "You need to . . . You should . . . You have to . . . eat."** I KNOW I need to eat, so you don't have to tell me over and over again. Plus, I'd like to eat when I'm hungry, not when I'm told. You make me feel like a baby when you say this, and seem to think I have no idea that a human needs food to survive. It's obvious. I also know I don't always eat on your calendar, but I'm trying. Just don't assume I should eat when you do. Besides, if I don't eat, maybe I'll learn the lesson without having you tell me like I'm an idiot.

As you can probably see, many of these common mistakes usurp your child's power, intelligence, and sense of safety. They create a silent power struggle between the parent and child that's not intended but actually fuels the fight, flight, or freeze response inside the child's limbic system, which translates to immune system over- or under-activeness. So, I leave you with the following tips:

- Remember, your goal as a parent is to nurture your child's sense of autonomy and control over the illness.

- You are shepherding a human being into adulthood. These years are their training grounds for childlike exploration, wonderment, and preparation for an emotionally regulated, self-sufficient adulthood.

- Autonomy is the beginning step toward feeling a sense of control over the illness, and to a child making their own decisions, which leads to fewer feelings of being helpless and incompetent.

The Top 5 Things to Never Say to Your Child With an AI or GI Condition

When raising children—whether sick or not—our words matter. The goal of this book is to help you empower your child to heal. That means there are some words and phrases that just don't support that goal. Why? Because we need to understand that what we say affects our children's limbic system: fight, flight, freeze, or faint. We need to avoid certain words, which I reveal in this chapter, so we can encourage our children's parasympathetic systems, which helps them "rest and digest."

The power of words to hurt or heal is real. It's called *neurolinguistic programming* (NLP), and it affects psychoneuroimmunology and healing. In the intricate web of mind–body medicine, the language we use has profound implications for health and healing. NLP, and its relevance to psychoneuroimmunology, sheds light on why words matter so significantly when dealing with disease, especially gastrointestinal (GI) and autoimmune (AI) conditions.

NLP is an approach that explores the relationship among neurological processes (neuro), language (linguistic), and behavioral patterns learned through experience (programming). Developed in the 1970s by Richard Bandler and John Grinder, NLP aims to understand and change human behavior through the power of language and thought patterns.[1]

The language we use shapes our beliefs, attitudes, and behaviors. Positive language can reinforce positive beliefs and promote healing. *Negative reframing* is an NLP technique that involves changing the way we perceive a situation by altering our language and thoughts about it. For example, the word "vomiting" may be attached to a fear of it. Changing the word to something more lighthearted, like "upchuck," may reduce the fear dynamic. Some words have intense emotional charges that when spoken can re-create or reinforce negative memories and emotions associated with them. Then, the body has physiological reactions to them as well. If I repeat a hateful word over and over, it will begin to trigger emotions that affect the body. For example, racial slurs can influence a person's state of peace and simultaneously signal the limbic system to fight, flee, or freeze. Simply put, words matter.

One therapeutic technique to reorient the meaning of emotionally charged words is called *anchoring*. The strategy involves associating positive emotions with specific triggers—or anchors—such as a word or gesture, to help manage stress and anxiety. For example, one can use funny words to replace triggering ones. I had a patient who had fears of choking to death. If I asked him about "choking," he felt like choking, and choking is all he ever thought about; asking about it made it worse. Instead, I asked him to come up with a name for the fear. So he named it "Jimmy." I would ask, "How's Jimmy?" He would laugh and say that Jimmy is losing power. Simply changing the word association helped him overcome his fear. Words matter, and so do the memories associated with them.

Numerous case studies have highlighted how individuals with chronic illnesses, including GI and AI conditions, have used NLP and positive language to improve their health outcomes. Parents can model positive language and self-talk for their children, helping them develop a more optimistic outlook on their health and life. On the basis of my own work with more than 100 pediatric patients, I can verify how important it is to be aware of what NOT to say. The words we use, both spoken and unspoken, wield immense power over our health and well-being. NLP and the field of psychoneuroimmunology offer valuable insights into how language and thought patterns can influence the mind–body connection, particularly in managing GI and autoimmune conditions. By harnessing the power of positive language, reframing negative thoughts, you can empower your children to heal more effectively, so here are Top 5 things to never say to your child.

1—"I understand."

To be candid, you don't understand, and there is no way you could. Even if you have an AI or GI condition yourself, you still don't understand. You are not a child or teenager living in a modern-day, high-pressure society suffering from an illness that feels like your body is betraying itself. This statement, even as you are trying to console your child, breeds resentment. Its invalidating and leaves the child feeling alone and isolated and as if they have not been heard. It inhibits them from expressing themselves and makes the suffering about you, not them. Instead, you can say, "I am here for you in whatever capacity you need me. I can listen, offer advice, or just sit with you. Which do you prefer? I can never understand all you are going through, but I will always stay by your side; we are in this together."

See the difference? Now, you're an ally willing to support them. Plus, you're empowering them to tell you what they need or want from you.

2—Stories about "back in your day" or how you once struggled.

The fastest way to get an eye roll and to elicit repressed anger they can't express is to talk about what life was like for you and how much you can relate (see Chapter 6). Although you're trying to demonstrate empathy, I will reiterate: You cannot relate, and no amount of past stories of all you overcame will achieve the outcome you are looking for—to relate to your child. Their brains are hardwired to be different from their "tribe," your family. If you bring up examples from your life, it becomes clear you are talking about yourself and not about them. They see this as negating their reality compared to your archaic parental reality, which breeds anger, resentment, and isolation.

Instead, say something like, "Tell me what it is like for you; I can't even imagine how difficult this is," or "What can I do in this moment to help you? How can I help you feel safe at this moment?" Even if you get the reply "Nothing," you will have created space to activate their parasympathetic nervous system's rest-and-digest response instead of their sympathetic nervous system's limbic fight–flight–freeze response. Little moments like these add up.

3—"You need to eat."

This comes up frequently, both as something kids wish their parents knew (see Chapter 7) and as things to avoid saying. So, let me emphasize that obviously, they need to eat. They know it, you know it. As adults, when we are told this, we have the rational mind to consider the advice. But a teenager? This sets off alarm bells, anger, and feelings of being out of control. The teenage brain is hardwired to begin to leave the tribe to avoid tribal inbreeding, so they are neurobiologically designed to defy us. The second you tell someone, especially a teenager, "You need to," you are usurping their power and autonomy in their minds. Imagine your spouse or boss always telling you need to meet your deadline, you need to turn in your report on time, you need to check your email, you need to cook dinner, and so on. "You need to" creates a defensive subconscious and muted fight response in most humans above age 10. Even if it's true, that they do need to eat, it still ignites a struggle for power and control over what they put in their mouths.

Instead, you can say, "What can I make for you to eat?" or "Hey, have you had any nourishment today?" "Are you able to keep any nutrients down?" "What time can I expect you to eat by?"

You can also ask your child to make a list of "safe" foods that they would like, and always have some in the house. Then ask, "Would you like to make the snack (or meal) or would you like me to . . . ?"

Another great tactic is to involve your child in grocery shopping. I have found that children who partake in shopping gain awareness of the process, learn what foods they like, see the investment, and appreciate the meals more. They may even cook their own meals, or help the parents with making meals. This helps empower children, increases their self-efficacy, and fosters a sense of well-being. We practiced this with my daughter when she was skin and bones, with no appetite. She gained so much pride in shopping for her meals, even shopping online. Her appetite magically improved as she felt empowered to help make decisions and be involved in the shopping process and in creating her own meals. Now, she loves meal-prepping for the family and is taking the lead chef role in the house. We can see her beaming with pride in her sense of accomplishment.

4—"Maybe it's in your head" or "It's a mental health thing," or "You have anxiety."

Odds are your child has anxiety, and odds are you or another parent does, too. Managing their emotional health becomes as critical as addressing their physical symptoms. Why is it important to not label a child as having anxiety outright? Anxiety is a multifaceted response that involves both emotional and physical elements. It can be described as a state of worry, fear, or unease about an imminent event or something with an uncertain outcome. Symptoms can range from restlessness, irritability, and difficulty concentrating to physical manifestations, like increased heart rate, muscle tension, and digestive disturbances.

Labeling can have a detrimental impact on your child's self-perception. Telling a child they have anxiety can lead to self-labeling whereby the child identifies primarily with the condition. So, now they are the sick kid with anxiety, which forms their identity. "You have anxiety" is also self-limiting, defining, and descriptive, and can become woven into the tapestry of their personality and health. This can affect their self-esteem and create a sense of helplessness.

Anxiety carries a stigma that might make the child feel different or flawed, which can exacerbate feelings of isolation and stress. Overemphasizing anxiety can shift the focus away from managing the physical symptoms of their GI or AI condition, leading to neglect in other areas of their health care.

I don't believe anxiety is an isolated emotion. It's a physiological state of being, a result of a thought or emotion that based in fear and a sense of helplessness and of being overwhelmed. Anxiety is a complex interplay of emotions and the physical manifestation of those emotions. Children believe what labels we give them and what we tell them about themselves. It's like giving them a crystal ball and telling them they are doomed for life—which nurtures more anxiety. Instead, try saying, "I can see you are struggling, feeling overwhelmed. Let's find a way to work through this moment in time." It's important to take a holistic approach, addressing both the physical and emotional aspects of the child's health without overemphasizing any single aspect.

Here are a few more tips:

- *Language matters.* Use language that normalizes their experience and focuses on coping strategies rather than diagnostic labels, for example, "Everyone feels worried sometimes, and we can find ways to help you feel better."

- *Thought patterns.* Anxiety often stems from negative thought patterns and cognitive distortions, such as catastrophizing or excessive worry about the future. Telling your child they are anxious reaffirms their fears and lays the blueprint that this is their life and future. Think of it this way: When you are upset, do you want your partner or your parents to tell you "Calm down"?

- *Confirmation of emotional fears.* Fear of pain, uncertainty about their condition, or worry about the impact of their illness on family dynamics can contribute to their anxiety of being a burden on the family. This increases anxiety, and in turn they worry how their emotional state is negatively impacting you, which exacerbates the initial response.

5—"You're strong," or "You can do this," or "Be brave."

Telling a sick child they are strong may seem supportive, but it can sometimes have unintended consequences and thus backfire. The child can believe the parent is saying this because they are actually weak and that the parent is trying to manipulate their truth. Here are a few more reasons to avoid these kinds of phrases:

- *Intention versus impact.* Although telling a child they are strong is meant to be encouraging, it can sometimes place undue pressure on them to live up to that standard, especially when they are struggling.

- *Perceived expectations.* Children might interpret "being strong" as needing to hide their pain, fear, or vulnerability, which can prevent them from expressing their true feelings and seeking the support they need.

The notion of strength may place an emotional burden on them in the form of a perceived pressure to perform, to always appear brave and resilient, which can be exhausting and isolating. Children may fear disappointing their parents or caregivers if they show signs of weakness, which can lead to suppressing their emotions and increasing their stress levels. I see this often.

Your child does NOT want to have to be strong all the time. Telling them they are strong, or brave, puts pressure on them to be. The truth is they may feel scared, weak, vulnerable, and unsure, and they want someone to make them feel better. They DO NOT FEEL STRONG, so telling them they are causes internal conflict. Constantly striving to be "strong" can contribute to mental health issues, such as anxiety and depression. It's crucial to encourage the healthy expression of emotions. Authentic resilience comes from the ability to acknowledge and work through difficult emotions, not just from presenting a facade of strength. Children have a subconscious pressure to be strong; in reality, they are clueless and helpless. They feel like a failure when they are not brave and strong for their parents because most children are people pleasers. I'd rather you validate how they truly feel.

Instead of focusing on strength, use language that validates the child's experience. Phrases like "It's OK to feel scared" or "You are doing your best, and that's enough" can be more supportive. Use affirmations that balance encouragement with empathy. For example, "I am here for you, no matter what" or "We will get through this together" provide support without pressure. This highlights their efforts, not outcomes. Recognize the child's efforts and perseverance rather than labeling them as strong. This approach focuses on their actions and coping strategies, which can be more empowering. By focusing on empathy, validation, and balanced affirmations parents and caregivers can provide more effective and supportive encouragement.

It's crucial to create an environment in which children feel safe expressing all their emotions and vulnerabilities. This approach fosters true resilience and emotional well-being, which are essential components of the healing process. By rethinking how we express support, and using the power of words thoughtfully, we can better empower our children to navigate their health challenges with confidence and emotional strength with authentic resilience.

Part 3

Becoming a Wellness Warrior

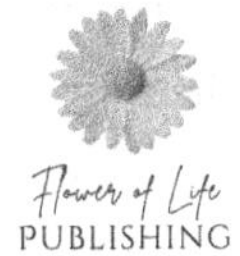

Chapter Nine

Your Child's Healing Phase(s), Part 1

UNDERSTANDING THE DYNAMICS OF THE MARTYR AND THE VICTIM

Does this, in one way or another, sound familiar? "Ugh (deep sigh). I'll just do it myself. No one understands how hard I work, all the sacrifices I make for this family. I bust my hump every day to provide for this family, and no one appreciates me. You all sit around watching television all day, talk on the phone and do nothing. *I* built this house for you all. *I* buy the food you waste. *I* pay for your lifestyle, and you all feel entitled to it. Then I have to do the dishes in the sink after I get home from work, while you all just sit there on the couch and ignore me. Fine, I'll do it. . . . Because no one else will."

If this does sound familiar, you're not alone—even if it's to a much lesser degree. This real-world example reflects the Martyr phase. You and/or your child may exhibit characteristics of a Martyr at some point in the healing process. In this chapter, I explain the various healing phases—Martyr, Victim, Survivor, Thriver, and Warrior—so you can identify where you (and your child) are, and where you want to be, as well as how to move from one phase to the next. I focus here on the Martyr and Victim phases and address the Survivor, Thriver, and Warrior phases in Chapter 10.

The example above came from a father who operates with an avoidant attachment style that has contributed to his daughter's autoimmune (AI) disease, which was affecting her optic nerve. The martyrdom energy in the quote is palpable and, unfortunately, contagious. The Martyr thinks other people are responsible for their unhappiness, hardship, and mistreatment—not them. Martyrs believe that because they sacrifice so much, other people must agree with them.

What the father did not acknowledge or relate to was the 2.5 hours the mother had spent driving their three kids around for all their activities and sports, the doctor visits she had taken them to, the snacks she had packed, the nursemaid she had played for the injured knee at soccer practice and the crocodile tears she had wiped away; the load of laundry she threw in at 5:00 a.m. so someone had clean volleyball shorts by 7:00 a.m., the grocery shopping, the dinner prep, and all the million other things that glue the home and family together. So, when the father comes home from work all he sees is a lazy (exhausted) family on the couch having some cuddle time after a long day, he takes it personally. He feels they are ignoring, and not appreciating, him. His Martyr energy clouds his judgment and ability to communicate in a safe, healthy manner. The result is that he avoids the family, dismissing any reality other than his own. Sadly, this father has been estranged from his adult children for years.

This mixture of an Avoidant parenting style coupled with a perpetual state of Martyr energy is an extreme case. But it provides an example of what we all have thought or felt at one point. We all have played a Martyr role and displayed passive-aggressive behaviors at some point. But imagine the emotional pain and discomfort this entails for a child growing up with this stress contagion. Between the parents spreading the emotional contagion, chronic invalidation (which, as research has shown, leads to disease),[1] an avoidant attachment style, and their progression through the various healing phases, is it any wonder why the child's disease process is being triggered? Regardless of your child's diagnosis, we as parents can observe with gentle curiosity how our patterns and behaviors affect our child's emotional safety and home environment.

Over the past 20 years of working with trauma, stress, anxiety, abuse, medical illnesses, and somatic illnesses, and having healed myself, I have come to formulate the five phases to healing, which I've experienced as well. A person can pass through these phases any time, and a particular phase can become more pronounced depending on life's stressors, work problems, job loss, trauma, family or relational issues, illnesses, or anxiety—or even when life is relatively simple and going well.

A married mother of one child comes to mind. This stay-at-home mom came from a place of privilege yet still had a cleaning lady. But the mom complained about all she had to do to ensure that the groceries were delivered and how she sacrificed her time away from playing Bunco with friends, as she drove her child to and from the neighboring school and cooked for three people. This was the role she asked for in her marriage, yet she played the suffering Martyr.

Healing phases are present even when life is seemingly good. So, when you read this chapter, you can read it from two perspectives: "What phase am I in?" and "What phase is my child in?"

The Martyr

A person who is going through the Martyr phase can be described as one who neglects their own needs, hopes, and dreams in order to serve others, the task at hand, or the family. This can be done in a helpful, kind, eager-to-please-others way or, like the father described earlier, in an angry, passive-aggressive way. With Martyr energy, the person feels like everything will fall apart if they aren't there to hold it together. They are responsible for everyone else's well-being and happiness. People in the Martyr phase will lack proper self-care, placing helping others above their own health and care by frequently sacrificing their own needs. They have difficulty saying no or setting boundaries, and they regularly work above and beyond set working hours.

You can think of a Martyr as a "noble sufferer" of sorts who willfully agonizes in the name of love, recognition, attention, or sacrifice while creating a space of awkwardness and discomfort for those around them. You feel as if you are walking on eggshells around them, but you don't know why. This phase is elusive yet definable, helpless and manipulative. I am no stranger to the Martyr phase; a lifetime of generational training helped me perfect it.

I recall that back when I had active multiple sclerosis, I had a service dog named Blu while I was attending undergraduate school at Southern Utah University. Blu was a blue-eyed Border Collie who was good at his job. He braced me when I couldn't hold myself up, and he helped me off the ground if I had to take a knee, which I did often when my legs went numb or I needed to lie down. I was an overachieving scholar, winning research awards and striving for a career in psychology. I excelled in terms of grades and completed unique research projects outside the scope of the graduation requirements. I traveled to speak at conferences to feature my research, which focuses on the concept that guilt is not an emotion. All this time, I took daily injections for my treatment; the prognosis didn't look good. My mentality was to fight back and beat the disease no matter what (note the anger and fight response in my mindset, perpetuating the limbic survival response). After taking a semester away from school, I went back because I believed I'd lose my cognitive abilities if I did not. I thought, *Why not go back to school and get my degree so I can keep my mind from declining more?* Unfortunately, the brain fog was real. I recall watching an episode of Seinfeld and not being able to follow along and understand the show. I stopped watching television because it confused me so badly. I became depressed.

I was also a Martyr. I was eager to please my professors, and my family, to prove I was important while perpetuating a chronic stress-related limbic response and a fight (not flee or freeze) mindset.

While working on research review boards, and serving as a teaching assistant, I did yet another extensive research project about religiosity and guilt. The work took months to complete and present at conferences, all in addition to my other school- and home-related workloads. My daily words and actions wanted recognition for all I was sacrificing. I loved Blu, but he was a crutch to show the world, "See, *I am* sick, I have a dog to prove it." An AI condition is a silent sickness, but I had Blu to show for it. I wanted the world to know how sick I was, and how much pain I had, along with all the sacrifices to make myself and my life mean something. I complained about all I had to do and did not have time to properly care for myself amid all my obligations. Who knew that would be the training grounds for this book?

The Martyr was a deeply subconscious role that played out my life. I had an inner desire that was driving me to justify my illness. It was as if I were saying, "Look, see all I can do, all I sacrifice. I am willfully suffering. No one expected me to do extra research, serve as a teaching assistant and on review boards. No one even asked me to go back to college."

Martyr was the first of five healing phases through which I'd wax and wane until I found my seat in the (silent) Warrior phase and repurposed my pain. I can catch myself now if I start noticing a Martyr or Victim attitude in myself. Those two phases carry a lot of emotions: guilt, despair, repressed anger, resentment, and stress, but mostly fear of losing control. All of these emotions are contagious.

People with anxiety, AI, and gastrointestinal disorders can get stuck in this overachiever–martyr bidirectional loop. One feeds the other at the expense of the child's health. If you recognized that your child is in the Martyr phase, it's important to understand why. A Martyr is not done being sick, not at all. There are secondary gains being met: maybe sympathy, a fear of slowing down, a fear of failure or disappointment, a fear of actualizing emotions, a fear of not pleasing others. A Martyr is intent on proving that they are a fighter who can beat the disease. Their pain serves a purpose—until it is repurposed for a greater outcome.

One key note to remember from this chapter is that it's not your job to try to change or address the phase of healing your child is in. This is not a conscious choice of theirs. These phases involve subconscious behaviors that are related to a number of factors. So, do not call your child out as acting like a Martyr. This will only guarantee an argument and defensiveness, and they will double-down and possibly get sicker. Instead, observe and understand what needs this phase is meeting for them. For example, are they trying to prove something? People-please? Are they operating out of fear of not being good enough? Or do they resent being sick?

A common driving force, which I know all too well, is the sense that their body is betraying them, and acting like a Martyr is their way of fighting back to beat the disease and regain a sense of control over their anxieties. I firmly believe that each phase serves a purpose, and I am so grateful for my martyrdom days. It taught me what passive-aggressive behaviors feel like and that gentle observation was a large part of my healing journey. Remember, feeling like a Martyr (or Victim) is very normal when a person is diagnosed with a serious health condition. But we don't have to stay stuck in that healing phase.

Without therapy, psychoeducation, and the development of self-awareness, the average child has limited inclination toward, or awareness of a particular healing phase or why they are in it. But please know, it is serving a purpose. Removing a purpose before they are ready has adverse effects. Instead, try to learn and understand their automatic negative thoughts and the secondary gains that are perpetuating this phase.

I know how frustrating it is for parents who want to step in and force their child to move on to the next healing phase. I've seen it in my own child and can relate. I had to embrace each phase, knowing my role was to love and learn, not fix them. I've seen the damage in my clients that resulted from parents who did not do this, and I didn't want the same outcome for my daughter Ella, as she struggled. So, I embraced her need to be exactly where she needed to be, with no judgment, even if it was very aggravating to witness at times. Ella spent about a year or so vacillating between the Victim and Martyr phases as she struggled to have her deepest needs met. I had to sit tight and empower her from the sidelines.

The Victim

The Victim phase can sometimes be confused with the Martyr mindset. They are similar, but there are significant differences. Victims take things personally. Even if a comment or statement wasn't directed at them, they believe it is. A person with a martyr complex will often go out of their way to take on extra tasks for other people, even if they don't want to. Martyrs want to please others, or seem like they are the only ones who can do a particular task, whereas Victims remain inactive out of self-pity.

A person in the Victim phase may feel like they have little control over or impact on external factors in their life, and that ongoing emotional pain leads to learned helplessness, a behavior pattern in which the person stops trying anything new because they are certain failure is inevitable. This learned help-lessness reflects what can happen as a result of the Helicopter and Bulldozer parenting styles. When parents complete tasks or remove obstacles for their child, although their intentions are good, the resulting cycle of feeling helpless and guilty conditions the child further into the Victim phase. This juxtaposition leads to a challenging proposition for the parent: How do you help your child suffer less without conditioning them to become dependent on that help?

This starts with communication that empowers. I'll discuss this further as the book unfolds, but here's an example.

My daughter Ella spent many months in the Victim phase. I would watch her from a distance and monitor her emotion regulation. It was like watching a volcano make a decision to explode or not: The slightest change in temperature could be catastrophic for all involved. , this could mean an emotional meltdown of epic proportion followed by days in bed with joint and spinal pain from the aftermath. (Side note: You may notice a pattern in which, one to three days after an emotionally stressful event, your child may get sick. It's an insidious cycle of emotion dysregulation and sickness, a seesaw, back and forth, and no one is in control.)

When I would see her get overly stressed with a task, I would ask, "Would you like my help? I trust you can figure it out and can ask for help, so I'm here *when* you need me." Some tasks would be just too much. It's like the person has one too many tabs open, and opening another tab causes the computer to crash. There is simply no mental and emotional bandwidth for extra tasks on some days, and that is OK. During these epic meltdowns, which happened on a daily basis for a long stretch, I would remind myself that her 14-year-old brain was not wired to handle a devastating potential future. She did not yet have a fully developed brain, so processing a sense of loss of the self before her self had even formed was unimaginable. The point I am trying to convey is that we should have compassion for people in the Martyr and Victim phases. They are experiencing indescribable fears related to facing a lifetime of anxiety and illness.

People in the Victim phase feel utterly out of control, that life is not fair, which breeds bitterness about the world they live in. They feel like their bodies are betraying them. With utter helplessness, and no one to blame, they may attack and blame others. They feel miserable physically and emotionally and have a deep sense of loss, anger, and sadness, feeling a tense hopelessness each day. This mental and physical anguish makes them ask daily, "Why me?" a question that is often followed by an empty silence. Even worse, they may think, believe, or say, "God is punishing me," with a sense that they are being punished for a perceived misdeed. That is another book in itself; religious guilt was the focus of one of my undergraduate research projects.

With Ella, the Victim phase led to emotional meltdowns because she needed reassurance about and validation of her pain and fears. She became hospital bound and homebound, and she had to be homeschooled because she was missing so much school. (I'll address this topic in Part IV, "The Balancing Act.") I knew the meltdowns and personal attacks were a cry for help and validation. She wallowed in a sea of self-pity, and she actually needed to feel that emotion.

This was not the time to be a toxic cheerleader and push her to "fight back" and "beat this disease." That would only create MORE pressure to get better, and it would be extremely invalidating of her pain and experiences.

The Victim already feels like a burden in many ways, and internalizes an immense pressure to "get better." Just because I didn't want Ella to suffer, I was not going to push my agenda on her to alleviate how painful it was for me to see her like that. As parents, we want to take ALL the pain away from our children and make them feel better. However, when they are in a Victim phase, supportive silence is powerful! Toxic cheerleading, telling them simply to "fight through it," teaches them that they can't trust you their darkest moments. Sometimes they just need to be held and told, "It's OK you feel this way. I'm here for you; as a team, we will figure this out." After telling them this, be silent. See how powerful silence is when they are suffering. Hold the space for just them, their experience, and you will be amazed how much your child will eventually open up to you.

I like to describe it as this. They are the cool kids in high school. We, the parents, are the nerds trying to sit with the cool kids at lunch. We can try too hard to just be around them.

Silence affords your child the space and time to decide whether they feel safe enough to be vulnerable and authentic with you to invite you into their world. If we as parents negate the Victim phase, they may spend years in it to gain the validation they are seeking and, in the process, prolong the sickness. We don't want them to suffer, but telling them they shouldn't feel a certain way will make matters worse. They are in fact suffering to some degree. This is their reality, and toxic positivity will only make it worse.

The days Ella did go to school, on rare occasions it hurt too much to walk the large campus, so she asked for a walking cane. My heart sank, and in my head I was screaming, "NO! You don't need one; I see you skip around the house on good days!" But I used my clinical knowledge and knew what this was: She needed others to KNOW she was in pain. Her cane was my Blu. She picked out her walking cane online, and I ordered it the moment she did. She was so happy. She felt heard, validated and understood, and empowered. She had taken control over something to make herself feel better, and she felt empowerment in a helpless sea of distress. We even ordered stickers to decorate her cane, and after was all said and done she was smiling.

Her dad didn't think we should support getting her a cane, and said instead that we should encourage her to do exercise, yoga, and so on, and encourage her to get better, not worse. I knew it sounded ironic, but I explained to him that this will pay off in the long run. So, I told him, "After you initially validate that you're glad it's helping her, don't ever mention the cane again. Don't offer any negative attention about it—just pretend like it's not there."

This is called an *extinction* of the behavior. In this case, we paid no attention to the cane, validated that Ella needed it, moved on, and let this all play itself out. So many times I'd see her skip around the house without the cane, and I badly wanted to ask, "Do you really need the cane today?" But I knew better. She would have had a negative reaction that would negatively affect her progress. I just kept moving us forward, planning fun events and trips, hoping it would make a difference. One day, she left her cane at home after she began to drive. I never said a word, no one has, and the cane is now retired. Two-and-half years later, it all paid off. I smile each time I walk by the unused cane hanging by the door.

The challenge for parents is when they see incongruences in their child's progress — one day they seem well and the next day they are bedridden. But stick to the plan. There are no finite patterns to when your child feels good or bad when in Victim or Marty phases. It will fluctuate. Even when Ella appeared to not need her own Blu, we didn't harp on the cane. We empowered her to make choices she felt were best for her, but we had the final say. Today, she wears platform shoes and is receiving her associate's degree the same day she receives her high school diploma, at age 17. She managed to pull off graduating in the top 10% of her class. If you recall from Chapter 6, after the neurologist schooled me when she was in third grade, I never again checked her grades or harped on her. The meltdowns eventually disappeared. Recently, she started feeling overwhelmed with all that's required to apply to college, and she asked, "Mama, can you help me?"

This may sound benign, but it's progress. When she needs help, she asks. She's empowered that way, even if she needs a good cry and a warm bath with a cup of tea. Her cane has been hanging next to the door for 2 years now. She still needs knee braces on long days working in the theater department, but she has moved on to the Survivor phase. I see glimpses of Thriver peeking out from time to time. I asked her once about repurposing the pain (silent Warrior phase) and using her lessons to help others. Her reply was, "Not yet Mama; I'm not ready." My heart melts when she still calls me Mama, and even more so with the word "yet."

Chapter Ten

Your Child's Healing Phase(s), Part 2

MOVING TO THE SURVIVOR, THRIVER, AND WARRIOR PHASES

The Martyr and Victim phases are difficult, but the next three phases—Survivor, Thriver, and Warrior—deliver hope for healing in spades. As we parents learn to empower our sick child by addressing our own attachment styles, something amazing starts to happen: We watch our sick child change for the better. Even though they may slip back to Martyr or Victim phases from time to time, as they take ownership of their condition and responsibility for their behaviors, choices, and actions they will begin to shed those phases. We begin to see them acknowledge that they are surviving their condition, which is a bold new phase that leads to healing.

The Survivor

My daughter Ella has been in the Survivor phase for some time now, which I'm so glad to see. The major marker that differentiates Victim from Survivor is *accountability*, the practice of being held to a certain standard. Your child must learn to accept responsibility for their actions and understand that if they choose unfavorable actions, accountability brings consequences. When Ella felt heard, validated, and understood, she was able to disarm her "fight" limbic response and feel emotionally safe. She didn't need to fight for validation or to be understood any longer. She never suffered from chronic invalidation. She is now aware of and accountable for her role in creating, fostering, and contributing to either illness or wellness. This includes being accountable for her automatic negative thoughts (ANTs), limbic response, self-care, school–social life balance, and overall, her commitment to emotional sobriety.

The concept of *emotional sobriety* indicates that we can become addicted to our feelings. Therefore, part of the healing process is learning to let go of the Martyr and Victim phases (and related emotions and secondary gains). This letting go—emotional sobriety—offers a sense of being comfortable and present with all of your feelings, without judgment for any of them and without allowing emotions to define or control you. Realizing that you can have a particular emotion is healthy, but allowing that emotion to become a part of your identity is not healthy. You can feel an emotion and not become that emotion.

How can you help your child move from Victim to Survivor? By nurturing self-efficacy. *Self-efficacy* is defined as "an individual's belief in his or her capacity to execute behaviors necessary to produce specific performance attainments."[1] The completion of small tasks can be perceived as accomplishments to increase self-efficacy.

Author Nicole Celestine wrote a great article on PositivePsychology.com, explaining the "4 Ways to Improve and Increase Self-Efficacy."[2] Of the four ways, *mastery experiences*, was identified as the most powerful driver. A mastery experience occurs when we succeed at new challenges. For example, something as simple as successfully cooking a new dish may increase self-efficacy. This is because mastery experiences are based on "direct, personal experiences rather than secondhand accounts." This direct evidence of past successes builds confidence in our capabilities in the future. Plus, we experience a reward when we observe how the investment of time and effort yields positive results, which creates an expectation that we will perform well in other new situations.

With regard to Ella, her dad and I decided that we needed to prioritize self-efficacy, childlike wonderment, and social time over schoolwork. I knew that the power of increasing her sense of self, rediscovering her playfulness, laughing, and finding her purpose was the key to guiding her out of the maze.

Mastery experiences allow us to accomplish tasks we may not otherwise have attempted. For example, for a depressed, anxious child who is suffering pain and fatigue, building a garden and tending to the plants and vegetables is something they can see prosper and grow. Ask your child about a hobby or idea they have always wanted to pursue. For Ella, it was theater. So, we allowed her to prioritize theater and social connections over schoolwork. I was playing chess, not checkers, while aiming at a long-term goal. The worst-case scenario would be that Ella would have to repeat ninth grade. In light of her condition and healing process, I knew there is no school if there is no health.

With increased self-efficacy, children with anxiety, depression, and autoimmune and gastrointestinal issues learn they are far more than a diagnosis or a disease. Despite their condition, they begin to believe they are capable of achieving anything.

The shifts from Martyr to Victim to Survivor occur daily, in the form of micro-movements. Finishing small daily tasks (either wanted and unwanted, like making a bed, going for a walk, starting a hobby) can be the micro-movements that lead to macro-change.

As your child builds self-efficacy and flourishes with accountability they will begin to feel a sense of control, and even a small sense of empowerment, over their lives and emotions. Over time, you will see glimpses of surrendering, which leads to the Thriver phase.

The Thriver

When your child reaches the Thriver phase you may begin to observe moments of glimmer: micro-moments of joy or peace when a person appreciates simple things in their environment. These innate, spontaneous moments reveal that your child is breaking down the walls of their negative beliefs and finding enjoyment in the wonder around them. The term *glimmer* was coined by Deb Dana, a licensed clinical social worker who specializes in complex trauma. In her 2018 book *The Polyvagal Theory in Therapy*, Dana noted that glimmers aren't grand experiences. On the contrary, she says, "They're micro moments that begin to shape our system in very gentle ways."[3] This may include catching your child smiling when your dog runs across the yard, or noticing an amazing characteristic about being in nature, or an honest appreciation for a nice long hug from a dear friend or loved one. These glimmers cue their nervous system to relax and have a positive effect on their mental health. *Glimmers* spark positive feelings, whereas *triggers* spark negative ones.

Although moments of glimmer happen spontaneously, we can facilitate opportunities to experience them. You can make a concerted effort to spend time in places or doing things that nourish your child. This involves limiting screen time so they can be aware of the serendipitous occasions all around. This mindfulness practice brings them into the present and in touch with their senses. These tiny, seemingly insignificant moments when they feel joy, pleasure, peace, and gratitude represent major progression through the healing phases. Try spending time in nature, noticing the sights and smells, or arranging family time to play a game together, go on an adventure, or connect with people your child enjoys, or simply allow your child (and yourself) some free time with no responsibilities. Even your child's favorite meal or candy bar, or the anticipation of their favorite movie or playing with their pet, taking a warm bath, or listening to the rain can produce moments of glimmer.

When you experience moments of glimmers, and can point them out to your child, you can model what they look and feel like. Depending on their age, your child may get really engaged with the moment, or they may roll their eyes. But they will begin to see what you are doing over and over each day, and when you are not looking they, too, will have moments of appreciation. This way, you can spread the emotion contagion of peace and gratitude. When you couple this with micro-movements of self-efficacy, you have moments in the day when they won't feel like a sick kid.

Sometimes, my patients tell me, "Yeah, but I still felt sick the rest of the day after the *one* glimmer I had." My reply, after fully embracing the Victim mindset, is "Yes, you did feel sick the rest of the day, *and* you also had ten minutes of reprieve from feeling sick you otherwise would not have had. Ten minutes a day adds up over time." This begins to renew their brain. Because you model what this looks like, you will be surprised how contagious gratitude, joy, and peace can be. Plus, you'll notice less of a focus on the illness and more on the amazing moments of glimmer just waiting to be experienced.

The Warrior

This final healing phase is something to behold. No longer a Martyr, Victim or Survivor, the Warrior has moved beyond the Thriver's newfound ability to experience moments of glimmer. The Warrior seeks these moments out, relishes the connection to self and others with a childlike wonderment for the world, and understands that emotional safety creates wellness in the self and in others.

A (silent) Warrior has no need to go into battle. Their emotions are in check, and they quietly hold themselves accountable for their decisions and behaviors. Plus, they can capture their ANTs when they come marching out and turn them into automatic loving thoughts. They are aware of secondary gains, attachment styles, limbic states, emotional contagion, and glimmers versus triggers. Warriors are silently powerful; they feel no need to fight or flee. Instead, they can protect their peace and be at rest, with an inner strength that comes from knowing themselves.

The hallmark characteristic that reflects the Warrior phase is learning how to repurpose pain. Now grounded in a healthy perspective about life and their condition, they may be willing—or desire—to help others, tell their story, and create beauty from their ashes in other ways. They've broken through their mental barriers to experience and give meaning to their lives.

This concept is founded in a theory called *logotheory*. Logotheory, or "healing through meaning" in Greek, is a psychological theory developed by Viktor Frankl.[4] On the basis of his experiences as a psychiatrist, neurologist, and philosophy student, he formulated this meaning-centered approach. When I look at the Warrior phase, I see commonalities with Frankl's logotherapy, which is characterized by the notion of the freedom to choose how we respond to life and are personally responsible for our choices. The Warrior also is motivated to find meaning and purpose in life, to learn from their mistakes while being able to laugh at themselves with a sense of humor. Also, the Warrior exhibits a balanced conscience, having the ability to stand for what they believe in while having the margin to love others in the process.

The Warrior phase is not without issues. Life takes care of that for us. But the Warrior can see problems as opportunities and dig up strength when there used to be none.

We can't force any phase on our children, and at times the phases may appear to be fluid, continually changing from one to another. This is growth and a sign your child is finding their way to empowerment.

Chapter Eleven

The Privilege of Victimhood

DOES YOUR CHILD HAVE THE TIME AND RESOURCES TO FEEL SICK?

If your sick child does not progress through the healing phases, a troubling stalemate can occur. Whether consciously or unconsciously, they may choose to remain stuck in the Victim phase. In my work, I've seen this increase with today's modern age of device addiction, along with post-pandemic isolationism. But there are other possible reasons as well, when they have the privilege of becoming a long-term victim. I call this impasse *the Privilege of Victimhood*; it is highlighted by their ability to avoid *and* marinate in their own problems and their absence of gratitude.

Some children with anxiety, autoimmune, and gastrointestinal (GI) issues run around with busy lifestyles, overworked and overextended in the pursuit of grades, athletics, and performances, spending their lives overachieving and trying to be perfect. On the other hand are those who are retired overachievers, (who have accomplished so much and can no longer sustain perfectionism so they seem to retire from that way of life) have failed to launch, or were once happy-go-lucky children who are now silent and isolated. They transform right in front of your eyes as they age, which can lead to increased anxiety, illness, or exacerbations of their existing condition, at a minimum. The first wave of anxiety occurs around age 8 or 9. The second wave happens in middle school, which is disruptive; most parents hope it's just the awkwardness of middle school and that the child will grow out of it. Instead, by the third wave of anxiety, which hits in early adulthood, from 18 to 23, their physical condition has become almost unmanageable. The chronic stress related to their external environment and temperament evolution are precursors to GI problems, headaches, or inflammation.

You may notice your child rarely wants to leave their room. They stop communicating and doing the things they once loved. They stop doing pretty much everything but instead hang out in their rooms on devices. They may complain about no (in-person) friends, or tell you how much they miss doing the things that they love, or they just stop talking altogether. Sometimes, you just wish to see them smile and laugh and engage, but they spend most of their time in their room, locked away, maybe playing video games, reading, or doom-scrolling social media or YouTube. They seem like Eeyore from Winnie the Pooh: melancholy, down or depressed, and withdrawn. Once a vibrant, healthy, vivacious child, now they complain any time they do interact, and they may let their grades suffer. Yet they have all their physical needs met and then some. Despite having supportive parents; dinner on the table every night; and multiple devices, games, books, toys, even vacations—basically anything they could ever want or need they have—they behave (and believe) like they have the worst life ever. Their illness has caused them to withdraw, perpetuating anxiety and leading, at times, to a sense of entitlement.

One 23-year-old patient of mine had achieved a lot for her age yet found herself stuck in the Privilege of Victimhood. She had graduated from college and had a well-paying job. Outside of work, though, she spent her time dwelling on the negative aspects of her circumstances. She had a nice roof over her head and a great family and support system of friends. Her remote job allowed her to travel, if she wanted to, and she was already saving for retirement. Unfortunately, she also had an extreme sense that the world was not fair because she did not have a boyfriend; this manifested in severe depression and anxiety. Wallowing in her own self-pity, she spent all her free time looking online for a boyfriend and complaining that she never could find someone to date. Her entire sense of self and self-worth was based on whether she could find a boyfriend. She spent countless hours using online dating apps, and online gaming, so she rarely left her room. This resulted in many sleepless nights and of her doing the bare minimum at her job.

The truth is, she had the privilege of excess time to entertain her sadness and a failure to experience gratitude.

We live in abundance. I am not implying we don't have problems; we can have problems and still live in abundance. We can have problems living in a tent, hunting for food, and walking miles for water we must purify, and yet still live in abundance. If we have food, water, shelter, and a sense of safety, we live in abundance. But that concept is completely lost on today's society and children, and in particular those stuck in Victim mode.

There was a point in time during my darkest hours, years after the wheelchair days, when I naïvely positioned my trust and self to be on the receiving end of extreme financial abuse. All my personal and professional assets were subjected to fraudulent activity from someone I deeply trusted. In order for me to work, I had to borrow my friend's Internet access, because mine had been maliciously shut off, so I sat inside my car, in order to be HIPAA compliant, and conducted patients' sessions over my phone. I still managed to find gratitude and abundance that I was able to sit in a car that was mine, have Internet access, and be able to generate income *and* help someone! That day, I wrote in my gratitude journal, "I am SO grateful I was able to make enough money to put gas in my car and help someone else at the same time." Those dark days taught me what abundance is. I had nothing to my name, nothing but a sense of abundance and gratitude that was generated from within. My children were safe and healthy at their dad's house. I was safe and healthy, and to top it off, I had a few bucks to buy Taco Bell! I had to make my dog rice that week rather than being able to buy her dog food, which at that point was way too expensive. When you are placed in a position to find your authentic truth and what really matters in life, you often realize you are already living an abundant life and feel grateful for that abundance; you've found the foundation on which to build your life.

You can be in a dire situation and not feel like a victim but actually *be* a victim. It's all in your choice of perspective. We *get to* pay bills, we *get to* work, we *get to* go to school. We *get to* buy groceries.

Some of today's children are so privileged that they are enabled to lie around using their iPads or iPhones or other devices, playing video games and doing nothing but think about their own pain, stomachaches, headaches, neuropathy, chronic pain, anxiety, abdominal pain, disease, and other problems. With the privilege of being able to have a lack of purpose, coupled with excess time, they spend countless silent hours on woe-is-me energy, with no passion or direction.

This—trying to inspire someone to realize that change is only one decision away—can be very difficult. There are 86,400 seconds in one day; that means each of us has 86,400 chances to make a new decision. The Privilege of Victimhood flourishes in the presence of boredom, which is the utter inability to use one's imagination absent from distractions.

As mentioned in Chapter 6, scholars in the field of cyberpsychology research analyze the psychological effects of devices and how those devices influence brain development, mood, and personality. Their research has explored how our bodies are in a state of maladaptive de-evolution of the brain, the body, bone and muscle structures, and even skull malformations as a result of headsets. Don't believe me? Try searching online for "gaming body." I have seen this over the past few years with male patients caught in the Privilege of Victimhood who are addicted to online activity. Females more often present with body dysmorphia and constant comparisons of themselves with women in social media. Children who are exposed to excessive iPad, device, and phone use lack the ability to use their imagination and begin to experience a decrease in self-efficacy, and an increase in anxiety and depression, as well as a hard-to-break dopamine addiction.[1] Sadly, addictions can develop even in children as young as age 2, referred to earlier in the book as "sticky iPad kids."

Parents may feel compelled to use the "back in my generation" mindset, saying or thinking, "I never had iPads to play with. We'd have fun playing with a stick. If they only *knew* how rough *I* had it back in my day. *My* parents didn't give me all I ever wanted." But this type of approach will only perpetuate the unwanted behavior.

If your child fits into the category of retired overachiever, or failure to launch, has slipped into the abyss of anxiety-related health issues with no real understanding why, and/or has stayed in the Victim phase for a prolonged period of time, ask yourself, with gentle compassion, "Am I enabling this behavior in any way? If so, how?"

It's difficult for parents, because we want to say to our children, "You should be grateful for all that we do for you!" As you may have learned first hand, or from this book, this will only create more withdrawal, distance, and discord. One of the interesting facts about over-thinkers is that they are chronic "under-feelers." The more a person overthinks, the less they feel the presence of the moment. The more time that someone spends thinking, "My life is so bad," or

"Why me?", the more they feel bad. This is negative energy-in-motion. These thoughts lead to emotions that create disease.

Imagine if they, and we, spent as much time thinking about gratitude as we do about our pain and problems. How good would we feel? I call these *automatic loving thoughts* (ALTs); they are the opposite of automatic negative thoughts (ANTs). If we can replace the thousands of ANTs flooding our mind with ALTs, a new dynamic will appear. When positive energy-in-motion is present, life takes on new characteristics.

Here's a tip for expectant mothers, or wanna-be parents: If I could do it all over again, I'd imprint my children with ALTs, every chance I could—from in utero, to the day of birth, and every day thereafter.

When I ask my pediatric patients, "Do you think you would still have anxiety, stomach problems, if you had to live in Ethiopia and walk six miles to get a gallon of water, and six miles back, just to make a bowl of rice? Would you have time to sit and think about how miserable your life is?" Ten out of 10 times their answer is "No; I'd be too busy." Then I see the lightbulb go on in their brain, and we open the discussion to exploring how to shed the Privilege of Victimhood.

With good intentions, you may have played a role in your child's problem by enabling their withdrawal from life. Parents who try to force gratitude on their children may experience a backfire in the form of apathy, which can lead to the child getting even sicker.

How can a parent shift their paradigm?

Watching a documentary film with your child about people who survive with very little may help you both realize the privilege we have. You can also replace or limit screen time with opportunities to experience moments of glimmer. Invite your child to experience life from a new perspective; try painting, photography, or hikes in nature. Ignoring their plight subtly inspires them to take action. I offered more suggestions in Chapter 8. The best way, however, to influence your child is to model *authentic* gratitude for and appreciation of the finer things in life. "I am so grateful for this good meal." "I'm so grateful for this warm cup of tea." "I'm so grateful I get to go pay the bills." "I'm so grateful I was able to pay for our cell phones." "I feel so abundant right now in life, even with everything going on." "I'm so glad we don't have to live in poverty like those people in the documentary."

Remember, vibes are contagious. You may recall from Chapter 4 that the number one indicator of a child's happiness is the parent's happiness, primarily the mother's. So, don't tell them how they should feel. Instead, reflect on what gratitude looks like, and you'll be surprised that a grateful attitude is contagious.

Chapter Twelve

Deactivating the Limbic System

DISENGAGING THE FIGHT RESPONSE

Imagine turning around and seeing a bear less than 10 feet away from you. Immediately, your mind sends signals to the brain's limbic system to activate its survival mechanism. A decision process occurs in nanoseconds—you can't outrun the bear, and it knows you're awake, so there's no point in playing dead. The only option is to prepare to fight for your life. The mind floods your veins with cortisol, your heart increases its rate of pumping blood into your muscles, and all your senses become heightened. This is the fight response.

Ideally, the bear wanders off and your mind and body settle down. But what if your mind and body do not settle down? What if the external and internal pressures of life keep you in a chronic fight response?

In short, disease.

In fact, a vast number of mental and physical disorders result from chronic stress, including cardiovascular disease, cancer, anxiety, depression, diabetes, autoimmune (AI) conditions, and gastrointestinal (GI) problems, which are some of the most prevalent. Long-term activation of the stress response system can disrupt almost all of the body's processes. Clearly, our mind and body were not designed to live in a fight response.

So, what can we do about it? We prepare a peace treaty with ourselves to deactivate the fight response. Here's what I mean.

Understanding the fight response, what to look for and why, is crucial for effectively managing its impact on mental, somatic, and behavioral health, especially in individuals with GI and AI conditions. But the fight response's impact goes beyond GI and AI conditions and into behavioral and chronic illness as well. For example, the fight response can lead to multiple sclerosis

(MS), which can manifest with both physical and behavioral changes—in this case, unexpressed anger and rage. As I was healing from MS, my turning point came when I released a lifetime of hidden rage and anger. I am still working with my daughter Ella to release her anger after being exposed to an abusive role model (not her father; he is amazing). This built-up, unexpressed anger can either create the fight response or be a symptom of it.

So, the fight response has a profound impact on mental health, physical health, behavioral changes, and on the immune system. What is the fight response, exactly? It's one of the body's primary survival mechanisms, designed to protect us from perceived threats. This response is part of the broader fight, flight, or freeze spectrum, which activates the autonomic nervous system (ANS) during stress. The limbic system, in particular the amygdala, plays a crucial role in detecting threats and initiating the fight response. When the amygdala detects a threat, it sends signals to the hypothalamus to prepare the body for action. Emotional stress, automatic negative thoughts (ANTs), an anxious attachment style, unhealthy work, school or family environments, chronic invalidation, and perceived or real threats can trigger the fight response. For individuals with chronic conditions like GI or AI diseases, this response can be heightened because of ongoing health challenges and stressors.

The mental symptoms of the fight response have cognitive repercussions. The fight response increases alertness and vigilance, making the person more aware of their surroundings and potential threats. I've mentioned this before, especially in my podcast: Imagine a long-tailed cat in a room full of rocking chairs. That poor cat is on high alert, scared to move in any direction, but will fight back against a threat in an instant.

During the fight response, cognitive focus narrows, leading to tunnel vision whereby a person may see only the immediate perceived threat and not consider broader perspectives. They become hyper-focused on something—be it an object, a thought, or an idea—that seems inconsequential to others. It's like a dog with a bone that won't give it up or allow any distraction from it.

The most common mental symptom by far takes the form of intrusive thoughts. Repetitive, intrusive, unwanted thoughts about the threat can dominate the mind, making it difficult to concentrate on anything else. Intrusive thoughts can make up the 48,000 to 50,000 negative thoughts we have about ourselves each day. So, if we really boil this down further, thoughts can create a chronic, perpetual fight response. It's a vicious cycle.

The most common emotional reactions from the fight response are obvious: anger, frustration, and irritability. Someone may be quick to snap at others; seem cranky; act withdrawn; or give off harsh, intense vibes that the whole room can feel. They are difficult to be around because they often seem so angry and/or passive-aggressive. They may slam things down, or slam doors, and then claim nothing is wrong. Anger often acts as a guard dog for sadness.

A person in fight response mode will often exhibit aggressive behaviors, whether verbally or physically. This may include shouting, arguing, physical confrontations, and/or defensiveness. Heightened defensiveness, over the smallest of matters, can strain personal relationships and social interactions.

I once had a 26-year-old male patient with a thyroid condition, and when his wife asked him to call her back or return a text he usually would snap at her in defensive anger and demand to know why she would ask such an intrusive question. He was in a chronic fight response state; he also demonstrated hyperactivity, restlessness, and insomnia. Increased energy levels can lead to restlessness and difficulty sitting still, which often manifest as pacing or fidgeting. This patient would often pick at his fingernails with an unsettling energy. He would start a project and never finish it, moving on to the next one and leaving a disorganized mess of trash and piles of junk all over his home. It was as if his home were a representation of his mind: chaotic, unhealthy, and messy. When his wife asked him to communicate, he would lash out and claim he was too busy with work and all the projects around the house. The anger oozed out of him, and his emotion dysregulation left no room for his family to feel safe. A person who has a long-lasting fight response as a child can carry it over into adulthood, marriage, and work.

In the realm of mind–body medicine, emotional dysregulation and anger play a critical role in shaping our physiological responses and overall health. The fight response also entails somatic symptoms, including an increased heart rate. The body prepares for action by increasing the heart rate and blood pressure to ensure that muscles receive more oxygen and nutrients. It can feel like your heart is beating so fast it's going to beat right out your chest. Muscles may become tense and ready for immediate physical action, leading to stiffness and soreness if sustained over time. This may feel like an unexplained sore neck or shoulders. The most common symptom of the fight response is noted in breathing, which becomes rapid and shallow, and begins from the upper chest rather than in the form of a healthy, deep diaphragmatic breath. This can reduce oxygen intake and contribute to feelings of dizziness or lightheadedness. The body's focus on immediate survival diverts resources away from digestion, potentially causing symptoms like nausea, cramping, or constipation. Chronic activation of the fight response can suppress the immune function, making a person more susceptible to infections and exacerbating AI conditions.

A Better Way to Let the Air Out

Breathing is one of the fastest ways to deactivate the fight response, but there's a big distinction between what helps and what hurts.

Do you recall watching your newborn lying on their back, perfectly still, sleeping soundly, and the only thing moving was their belly? This deep, slow and rhythmic up-and-down pattern is called *diaphragmatic breathing*. This is very different from the short, choppy chest-breathing done when one is in a fight response.

As life's pressures accumulate, whether internal or external, how we breathe reflects how well we're regulating our emotions. Between peer pressure, social media, global wars, stressed-out parents, ANTs, attachment styles, schoolwork, and performances, there's a lot of potential to trigger a fight response. Chest breathing can either trigger a fight response or be a reflex demonstrating the fight response. The hallmark sign of chest breathing is short, choppy breaths. This occurs when the muscles between the ribs and the neck work hard to raise and lower the rib cage to pull air into the lungs and push air out of the lungs. Chest breathing requires more effort to move less air. The medical term *dysfunctional breathing* also refers to a group of disorders: paradoxical breathing (upper chest breathing), erratic breathing, breath holding, and breathing too deeply or erratically (i.e., a panic attack).

Our breathing changes in response to our emotions, , happiness, anger, anxiety or fear. Our breathing is influenced by a complex interaction between the brain stem and the limbic system. Respiration is important in maintaining physiological homeostasis, and it coexists with emotions. But when we experience perceived threats to safety or internalized stress, the mind and body react accordingly with chest breathing to prepare to fight or flee (i.e., the flight response.

Stress changes how we breathe, which affects the amount of oxygen we absorb. A lack of oxygen in cells contributes to the disease process. Chest-breathing patterns are useful in short bursts when running from danger. However, prolonged chest breathing can contribute to a number of physiological and psychological conditions. For example, when chest breathing becomes the default method, dysfunction occurs in the upper chest and the abdominal area.[1] This can contribute to gastroesophageal reflux disease, or GERD; asthma; tension and headaches; as well as anxiety and paranoia, to name a few.[2]

So, what's a better way to let the air out and deactivate the fight response? When it comes to the correct way to breathe, it doesn't matter whether you breathe through your nose or your mouth. It is *where* you breathe— from the chest or belly—that matters. Try breathing like a baby.

Research has indicated that people with GERD who practice belly breathing after eating reduce how often they experience acid reflux.[3] For those suffering from GI symptoms, diaphragmatic breathing offers specific benefits: Activating the diaphragm creates a gentle massaging action felt by internal organs like the intestines and stomach; this can reduce abdominal pain, urgency, bloating, and constipation.

Diaphragmatic breathing facilitates the activation of the parasympathetic nervous system (PNS), which can be thought of as the relaxation response of the body, or the rest-and-digest state. Diaphragmatic breathing can help in specific GI-related situations:

- *Diarrhea and urgency:* Diaphragmatic breathing can help calm the digestive track and ease those moments of panic (i.e., "I MUST get to the bathroom immediately!").

- *Constipation:* Diaphragmatic breathing can be used to calm and massage your digestive system while you are sitting on the toilet attempting to have a bowel movement. The result may be a more complete bowel movement.

Belly breathing also promotes a sense of calm relaxation. That's why it's typically part of mindfulness practices and yoga.

The functions of the diaphragm affect the whole body system. Belly breathing affects the gamma waves, which involve areas of the brain that are activated for cognitive function: memory, attention, sensory perception, problem solving, and language processes.[4] Belly breathing muscle memory will occur; we just need to retrain our bodies how to go back to this natural state.

I tell my patients of all ages, "Let's do 'stuffy breathing.'" Then, I demonstrate how to do this. Lie on your back, and place your favorite stuffed animal on your belly button. Now, raise the stuffy to the ceiling with your inhale, pushing it upward, moving only your stomach to the ceiling. This is like pushing for a bowel movement as you inhale. Then exhale slowly, slowly dropping the stuffy imagining that you are pulling in your belly button to your spine. Then, repeat. "Inhale, stuffy up; exhale, stuffy down." Stuffed animals make them laugh, and we can play and laugh only when we feel safe. The PNS is activated at playtime. Laughter and childlike wonderment are disarming at any age.

I've learned that now my patients will often carry their stuffies to doctors' appointments, on car trips, and even sneak them into their backpacks so they have this tool ready and waiting. "Stuffy breathing" becomes linked to feeling safe and calm. Some kids will reach into their backpacks to pet the stuffy just to remind them they are safe.

Another trick is to have your child pick a soft favorite material from a blanket or felt piece of cloth. Cut a pocket-size corner of the blanket so they can keep it with them when they feel unsafe and nervous. They can reach in and feel the soft piece of blanket, self-soothe, do their belly breathing, and say the mantra they created with me in therapy. Typically, it sounds something like, "I am safe. I got this." You can even apply an aromatherapy scent, like lavender or peppermint for nausea, to the cloth.

Emotions that get buried alive need to find a way out before we can connect to a calmer state. My favorite exercise is to have a child scream into and hit a pillow and write a "for their eyes only" letter. This is a rage-filled private letter in which they express all their deepest, darkest thoughts that is for their eyes only. They get to destroy this letter, so they should feel safe enough to let out their anger, knowing they won't get in trouble for expressing this anger on paper because no one will read it.

If you have your child write one of these letters, try to refrain from reading it. As tempting as it may be to read it, that won't be helpful unless you suspect someone is harming your child. If you do read it, which I do not recommend, be prepared. The letter may be about you, and telling your child that you read it will break their trust, and you risk them burying their emotions more, causing an even greater divide between you. If you have specific concerns, you can have your child write the letter and review the letter with their therapist. In my experience, I allow the child to express their anger and have the power to destroy the letter to let the deep, hidden pain out without concerns about judgment from others. Every time I have seen, or read, a single "for your eyes only" letter, the patient reports how much better they feel after getting their hidden rage out.

How I Deactivated the Fight in Me

When I recognized that I was continually putting my body into fight mode, I knew the responsibility fell on me to take accountability for that (survivor mindset). I started with being very mindful of where my breaths were coming from and checking on my own breathing every hour until I retrained myself to belly breathe all the time. Then, I took to the trails for my favorite activity—walking in nature. Walking in nature benefits our health in many ways, including disengaging the limbic responses. This activity opens our senses to the wonders around us—seeing flowers in full regalia, appreciating fresh pine scents, feeling the ground variations under foot.

Hearing the birds chirp while outside helps us, too, on a primal level. Birds are keenly attuned to their surroundings, singing only when the environment is safe. It sets off the subconscious cue that we are safe, too. Songbird tunes serve as a sign of peace and safety, tapping into our primal instincts and signaling our nervous system to relax, rest, and return to a place of equilibrium.[5] This helps distract our mind from feeling threatened, allowing us to settle into the environment.

Another method I use frequently is listening to binaural beats. A binaural beat is an illusion created by the brain when you listen to two tones with slightly different frequencies at the same time. Your brain interprets the two tones as a beat of its own. Binary beats are good for mental health because they have been linked to encouraging positive feelings.[6] Or create your own playlist of feel good, hand-selected music. This creates an opportunity for me to connect with God and self. I also go barefoot on grass and try to get early sunlight exposure for at least 10 minutes a day with no sunglasses on. There is so much research that supports the benefit of earthing and sunlight exposure. Connecting with the earth, barefoot, can reduce inflammation and stress levels, and sunlight exposure improves our circadian rhythms, improving sleep function.

Healing begins with a decision, forcing ourselves to do the things we don't feel like doing in order to feel the way we want to feel. If we wait to feel like changing, we may never change, so it boils down to a choice. This leads me to my all-time-favorite tool for limbic deactivation: cold water exposure. Cold water exposure helps deactivate the fight response. It's a practice that is becoming increasingly popular for its health benefits. It has profound effects on the ANS, particularly in deactivating the fight, flight, or freeze response.

Cold water exposure stimulates the vagus nerve, a major component of the PNS, which promotes relaxation and recovery. This activation counteracts the sympathetic nervous system's fight, flight, or freeze response. Improved vagal tone through cold exposure helps regulate the heart rate and promotes a state of calm, reducing the overall stress burden on the body.

Immersion in cold water can reduce systemic inflammation. This is significant because chronic inflammation is often associated with prolonged stress and the fight response. By reducing inflammation, cold water exposure can alleviate some of the physical symptoms of chronic stress, such as muscle tension and pain. Exposure to cold water triggers the release of endorphins, which are natural painkillers and mood elevators. This release can create a sense of well-being and reduce perceived stress levels. The increase in endorphins can lead to improved mood and decreased anxiety, helping to deactivate the fight response and promote a more balanced emotional state.

Regular exposure to cold water can increase the body's resilience to stress by enhancing its ability to adapt to new stressors. This process, known as *hormesis*, involves exposing the body to mild stressors for the purpose of building resilience. Over time, the body's improved stress response can reduce the intensity and frequency of the fight, flight, or freeze reaction in everyday situations.

Sunlight exposure, music with binaural beats, nature, birds, earthing or connecting to the earth barefoot, and cold water exposure all are evidence-based strategies to increase PNS activity. What's not included? Absorbing the daily news, reading nasty comments on social media, and watching scary television programming. I also started putting down all my devices about 2 hours before bedtime. The goal is to activate my rest-and-digest system with every choice. For me, dedicating my time, thoughts, and activities to regulate my nervous system became as important as my full-time job and raising my kids as a single parent. I knew the long-term consequences that would result if I didn't take regulation of my nervous system seriously, because healing cannot occur until my limbic system is deactivated.

This was also my first order of business with my daughter Ella, secondary only to her feeling validated by me, her dad, and the doctors. I knew that modeling what I wanted her to do, not telling her what to do, would be critical. I didn't want to be the kind of parent who operates from a "Do what I say, not what I do" approach. So, I showed her how to begin the healing process through my actions, breath work, and sharing what it feels like to feel at peace. As you know, mirror neurons and good vibes are contagious. So, I'd invite my kids to walk with me in nature or at a park to swing on the swing sets—sometimes I'd insist they join me too! We also created a new tradition of playing board games and cards at all family gatherings. Hugs are huge, and I give them at least twice a day, if not more. When we hug, the body produces the hormone oxytocin (also known as the "love hormone"), which is released from the vagus nerve. Hugs are important to social connectedness and safety. You may have 539 Facebook friends sliding into your DMs or commenting on your posts, but who hugs you at the end of the day is what matters.

I modeled cold water exposure with my girls when they were teens. They balked at me saying, "No way," when I asked them to try it. I kept up the practice for myself and didn't say a word to them for a while. Then, I threw out some one-liners about the benefits, only to get eye rolls from them as they changed the conversation.

One day, however, I had to force the issue with Ella. Her pain was so intense that she felt sick and nauseous. She was vomiting from the pain. Her choppy chest breathing was interrupted with stints of holding her breath completely. Her face turned red, then pale white from hyperventilating.

"OK, that's it. Ice bath now, and this is not up for debate," I demanded in my stern mom voice. She begged me not to. But I knew the cold plunge would stop this response, her panic attack and vomiting. I knew how neural pathways were forming at this moment that would imprint and train her brain to react with these negative symptoms again. It was tough love for sure, and she was not happy with me. I felt like Mommie Dearest for a moment. I put a towel over her so she felt safe, and I started the cold water in the tub and got ice from the freezer. I spoke calmly in a slow, soft voice while breathing from my belly so her mirror neurons would pick up the fact that this was not only safe but helpful. I guided her through the experience, telling her to focus on my eyes and slowly breathe from her belly, like I was doing.

Within just a few minutes, Ella's symptoms disappeared. She felt so much better! Afterward, I apologized to her for having to force the issue, but she totally understood because of how good she felt. That night, Ella slept for 10 hours and woke up feeling ready for the day. I never asked her to keep taking the cold baths. Two years later, she does cold baths weekly on her own. My other daughter, who does not have an AI condition, also takes cold showers just because she learned how good she feels and saw how much Ella and I love it. Silent modeling worked, with no nagging, no pressure. I lead with my own self-care, and they follow. These weekly cold baths help keep Ella's nervous system calm, along with her daily stretches and her version of meditating, which is putting makeup on. I'll take it in any form! She is calm and focused while doing makeup, and it makes her happy. She also enjoys painting, which is another great coping tool when she can't sleep.

Moments of a deactivated limbic system create neural pathways that build deeper grooves in the brain, resulting in new habits. We all have a few minutes every day to practice these methods to achieve a resting, calm state. So, make these moments count, and you will slow the growing up process to give them a chance at regulating their fight response in the future.

Landing the Flight Safely

Cultivating Safety When the Mind and Body Want to Flee

Panic attacks became as familiar as Monday mornings. Like anticipating the work week, I felt a panic attack coming when my gut started churning, heating my body temperature way above normal. I knew it was coming, and wanted to run from it, but there was no way out of my office setting. Feeling trapped, I couldn't focus on anything else except the most troubling symptom—sweat. Although I'd be sitting at my desk, my palms would literally drip sweat onto my computer. I knew I'd have the embarrassing moment of shaking my clients' hands soon, and the thought was daunting. Sweat would bead above my upper lip and drop from my forehead. Under my arms, my glands acted more like water sprinklers, soaking my shirts effectively. I came prepared, however, with special padded undershirts. But they'd turn into soaked underarm diapers within minutes.

Soon the moment would arrive. The meeting that hit my panic button. I didn't really have a reason to be so freaked out, but try telling that to my brain and body. With stomach churning, I'd feel nauseous. My bowels felt pressured, so I'd rush to the nearest bathroom to sit on the toilet, hoping that would relieve the panic and allow me to drive to the meeting.

Alas, for every client meeting, I'd arrive and before checking in, I'd visit the men's room again, pull a thick wad of paper towels and stick them under my arms. Then, I'd run my wrists under cold water, trying to cool down my body temperature. Plus, when I reached my hand out to shake, I could apologize in advance because "I just washed up."

During the meeting, I tried to smile and act as if I was the confident young man they had hired. When handed a sheet of paper, I tried to hold it as gently as possible so my fingers wouldn't leave sweat marks, but they always did. I couldn't raise my arms or the paper towels would fall through my sleeves. Besides, even if I wore a sport coat, I knew sweat stains would appear under my arms.

My partner, on the other hand, was cool as a cucumber. He enjoyed the meetings, which was impossible for me. He could focus on the conversation, while my thoughts swirled in overwhelming desperation. Oh, how I longed to be in swim trunks on the beach. But I was stuck, and all I could do was wait.

***

I asked a colleague to write the above after he told me about his previous experiences with panic attacks. For him, they came two to three times every day. This miserable mind–body experience is a perfect example of the limbic flight response, a survival mechanism that's engaged when we need to flee from trouble. Although his experience may be considered an extreme response, panic attacks are quite common, and anxiety even more so.

The flight stress response also has mental, somatic, and behavioral symptoms. Mental symptoms of the flight response are similar to those of the fight response, but often the thoughts are more fear and worry based. The flight response often involves a surge in fear as the mind focuses on escaping the perceived threat, how to avoid or escape a situation. Escaping the perceived threat brings a sense of relief. Intense feelings of panic and fear can dominate, making it difficult to think clearly or rationally. The mind may be overwhelmed with rapid, often repetitive thoughts about the need to escape or avoid the threat with an urge to flee.

Chronic activation of the flight response can lead to avoidance behaviors, whereby a person steers clear of situations that they perceive as threatening. This manifests with children by avoiding school or social situations. If they cannot avoid these situations, panic sets in.

When a flight response kicks in, a rise in heart rate follows, which pumps more blood to muscles, preparing the body for rapid movement along with rapid breathing. Breathing becomes faster and shallower, providing more oxygen to the muscles. Increased perspiration accompanies the panic response to help cool the body during the anticipated intense physical activity.

The body diverts resources away from digestion, potentially causing symptoms like nausea, stomach cramps, or diarrhea, as well as loss of appetite: The body's focus on survival can suppress appetite, leading to a lack of interest in food.

The two main behavioral symptoms of the flight response are avoidance and withdrawal. Children may physically remove themselves from situations they find threatening, sometimes abruptly leaving places or avoiding them altogether. Chronic activation of the flight response can lead to social withdrawal, as the person avoids interactions that may trigger anxiety.

Hypervigilance and constant scanning of the room are also common. A heightened state of alertness can lead a person to constantly scan their environment for potential threats. One of the most common manifestations of the flight response is the startle response. An exaggerated startle response, in which a person reacts strongly to unexpected stimuli, is common.

Irritable bowel syndrome (IBS), and diarrhea, are common flight response disease manifestations. One 17-year-old female patient of mine had a prolonged, chronic flight response and suffered years of unresolved IBS, nausea, loss of appetite, and diarrhea. She was diagnosed with cyclical vomiting syndrome (CVS).

CVS is one of my favorite conditions to treat because it can be cured so quickly and it's so rewarding for all involved. Rarely do I use the term *cure*, but for CVS a cure is in fact possible because it typically resolves in a matter of weeks. Plus, it can be clinically documented as doctors track when the vomiting cycle stops.

I have worked on the most fascinating cases of CVS as a prolonged flight response. When we are faced with danger, we either fight, flee, or freeze. Our bodies naturally expel whatever they can to make us lighter and faster to run and flee. For example, often the flight response will trigger a need to urinate or defecate, sometimes involuntarily. The fight, flight, or freeze response triggers a release of hormones that disrupt the usual hormones that keep the bladder relaxed, causing it to contract.[1] Another physical response to extreme stress or anxiety that can result is involuntary vomiting. Stress vomiting is primarily driven by emotional or psychological factors rather than physical factors.[2]

Stress vomiting is not a medical condition in itself but rather a physiological response to stress. When I work with patients with CVS or stress vomiting, I try to identify the initial sensitizing event (ISE), which is one major stressor that left a significant impact on the psyche, or its from previous trauma (and trauma is not the event that happened to us, but how that event stored in our bodies). My CVS patient, mentioned earlier, had her boyfriend pass away a year and half prior. She was very sick, in and out of hospitals. She was unable to keep food down and was vomiting bile and dry heaving. It was bad. After more than a year of having CVS, in cycles that lasted weeks at a time, only heavy anesthesia would alleviate the symptoms. Her family was desperate. She was ready to give up—not necessarily suicidal, but hopeless about living with this condition. Her mental health suffered. Although she loved life, gardening, and the outdoors, her condition had reduced her to kneeling on the bathroom floor hovering over the toilet for hours, days, even weeks at times. This is how she lived for a year; her life as a happy-go-lucky typical teenager had evaporated.

Once she and I had identified the ISE and the limbic flight response, we began to work to deactivate the limbic response. This included allowing her to grieve. It took about 1 month to stop the vomiting then another few months to process the grief.

Another CVS case was an 18-year-old freshman in college, named Lilly. I interviewed her on my podcast because her story is truly remarkable. Like many of my patients, she was an overachiever, pushing herself too hard to be perfect, please everyone, keep her college scholarship, and make her family happy. Her body began to retaliate from all the pressure, and she became stuck in a flight response as she subconsciously tried to avoid and escape all of her pressure to be perfect. Once we had identified this, she worked hard to deactivate her limbic system. It took 1 month of cold showers and walks outside before a noticeable difference was observed. Lilly schedules maintenance appointments from time to time as old patterns of perfectionism arise. She knows that when life gets too stressful, her body's default response is to vomit. She has learned to not attach anxiety to the experience, so she holds no attachment to her body's response. She knows how to recalibrate herself to return to homeostasis without attaching a mindset of freaking out, fear, or loss of control. She reframes her thoughts as *OK, I'm off balance, let's get back on track; this is temporary.*

If we incorporate mind–body practices, such as mindfulness, to our energy and interactions, belly breathing exercises, and replace automatic negative thoughts with automatic loving thoughts, we can help modulate the flight response, reduce stress, and enhance immune function. Through these integrative approaches, we can support the journey to healing and resilience, fostering a more balanced and health-oriented perspective for both our children and ourselves.

Chapter Fourteen

Melting the Freeze Response

REFRAMING THREATS TO AVOID A MIND–BODY SHUTDOWN

Ruthie, the miracle patient I introduced you to in Chapter 2, became stuck in a chronic long-term frozen immobilization response, which caused her vagus nerve to be flooded over time. Her mind was in a limbic state, frozen from prolonged trauma. Her biology was in limbo, frozen, unable to eat. Think of a fainting goat, playing possum, or a deer immobilized in front of a car's headlights as examples of the primal frozen response. A deer does not have the need to eat when staring into a car's headlights. The body may prepare for impact, and may urinate or defecate to lighten the body's load and thus increase the odds of survival, but overall the biological freeze presents as frozen biologics: constipation and bloating.

The part of the vagus nerve that is affected is called the *dorsal vagal nerve*. An immobilization or frozen response is initiated by the *dorsal vagal complex* (DVC). The DVC is a complicated, and brilliant, survival mechanism of the brain that activates the frozen response so we can avoid danger. In a frozen response, the body becomes numb to emotions in order to survive the environment.

The DVC limbic freeze response is more common than you would think. In this response state, you feel like you are walking around on autopilot as you go through the motions of life, with no emotions. Polyvagal theory provides a framework to understand the role of the freeze response in disease processes. Developed by Dr. Stephen Porges, polyvagal theory explains how the autonomic nervous system regulates physiological states and behaviors in response to perceived safety and threat.[1]

I have already discussed how the parasympathetic nervous system (PNS) promotes the rest-and-digest response, promoting a sense of safety, social engagement, calmness, and optimal digestion. This work is achieved through the *ventral vagal complex*. The opposing system is the DVC, which serves the limbic system's freeze response to extreme threats or prolonged stress, conserving energy by slowing down metabolic processes. These threats may include prolonged school stress, family dynamics, medical traumas, attachment styles, automatic negative thoughts, mass shootings, chronic invalidation, people pleasing, and overachieving; all of these are factors that contribute to external and internal pressures and expectations.

We all have a fail-safe survival mechanism in the DVC when the PNS spikes. Such a spike can come on so strongly that it overwhelms the sympathetic arousal and sends the person into a freeze state. This can take the form of a full collapse; dissociation (feeling disconnected from the self and the world); or a more partial freeze, such as an inability to think clearly or access words or emotions, feeling numb, doom-scrolling, not wanting to be around others, or not being able to move parts of the body. This can be momentary, short term—such as a possum freezing and becoming reanimated after the predator leaves or, in humans, it can continue indefinitely. A freeze state can happen in response to a real external threat or the perception of threat. Either fighting or fleeing can resolve the stress. However, if neither is possible or successful the sympathetic arousal can get so extreme that it is too much for the body to handle at this point, but we have a fail-safe survival mechanism: freeze.

Individuals with chronic anxiety may experience persistent activation of the freeze response, leading to feelings of numbness, detachment, chronic fatigue, fibromyalgia, widespread pain, bloating, and constipation. The freeze response can alternate with hyper-vigilance, whereby the person remains in a heightened state of alertness, anticipating danger. Chronic activation of the freeze response can dysregulate the immune system, contributing to autoimmune (AI) processes in which the body attacks its own tissues. Persistent stress and immobilization responses can lead to chronic inflammation, a key factor in many AI diseases.

The DVC's activation can slow or even shut down digestive processes, leading to issues such as IBS, bloating, gas and other gastrointestinal (GI) disorders. The gut–brain axis, which involves communication between the central nervous system, and the enteric nervous system (ENS), which is a complex network of nerve cells in the digestive tract that controls digestion and other functions. The ENS is heavily influenced by vagal tone. Disruption in this communication can exacerbate GI symptoms. If we have unresolved trauma, even medical trauma; or stuffed-down, unexpressed emotions; fearful–anxious thoughts; people-pleasing tendencies; perfectionism; a tendency to overachieve; and automatic negative thoughts (ANTs), we may live in a perpetual state of fight, or flight, or freeze. We may be able to channel this fight, flight, or freeze anxiety into activities such as cleaning the house, raking the leaves, working out at the gym, controlling our diets, excessive schoolwork or extracurricular activities, and work.

For some trauma survivors, however, no activity successfully channels their fight, flight, or freeze sensations; as a result, they feel trapped, and their bodies shut down. They may not be able to cry, or they may feel like they are on constant autopilot, numb, functioning like a robot, depressed but still functioning. The body prioritizes protection, lowering both mobility and arousal levels, as if preparing for a situation from which it cannot escape, almost like preparing for death. This might result in our feeling extremely tired, numb, or disconnected from both the world around us and from our own emotions. It's the body's way of shielding itself during overwhelming situations. Interestingly, this manifests as an outward appearance of calmness that masks significant internal disconnection and immobility. In contrast, one may vacillate among DVC shutdown, and hyperarousal, with conditions such as anxiety and obsessive-compulsive disorder, which tend to be more sympathetic dominant. It feels like this is a roller coaster of insanity but is simply the nervous system struggling for balance and a sense that one is safe.

If this response goes on for too long, it may develop into a more extreme version of DVC shutdown: fainting, also called *psychogenic syncope*, that is, an episode of fainting that is caused by psychological factors rather than purely physiological conditions. Psychogenic syncope is often linked to intense emotional stress, trauma, or anxiety. Symptoms include a sudden loss of consciousness; muscle weakness; and, unlike after an epileptic seizure, a return to consciousness without confusion.

Common triggers of psychogenic syncope also include overwhelming fear, panic attacks, traumatic memories, unexpressed emotions, anger, pain, toxic relationships, and unhealthy attachment styles. I have seen the partners and children of avoidant people and parents who neglect their loved ones' emotional needs struggle with psychogenic syncope.

In one case, a wife was very emotionally neglected. Whenever she spoke up to ask for a need to be met, even a simple one, her husband would verbally attack her for putting demands on him. He claimed that if she really knew him, she wouldn't be asking him to call or text her. She should just *know* he loves her; he shouldn't have to communicate that. She became too fearful to ask for basic communication, or simple needs to be met, and, in an extreme emotional shutdown response, began to pass out. She did not feel she was able to fight back and use her voice for fear or retaliation. She reported feeling stuck and overwhelmed. It was a tragic case of emotional abuse and trauma that landed her in the hospital twice. However, once she left the relationship, her health returned. Unfortunately, this is all way too common in unhealthy relationships, and the body will tattle-tale on the relationship even if the person won't. I have seen this in older teens as well; as soon as they leave the house, the syncope stops.

People with a history of anxiety disorders, post-traumatic stress disorder, or unexpressed emotions are prone to psychogenic syncope. Attachment styles and the way one receives love and validation play a significant role in DVC shutdown. In every case of psychogenic syncope I have ever worked with, the loved ones were shocked their child or partner had been silently suffering in so much pain.

In summary, the mechanism of psychogenic syncope, subsequent to the activation of the DVC, occurs in situations of extreme psychological stress, emotional invalidation, emotional neglect, or trauma. The brain perceives a threat that activates the limbic system, in particular the amygdala. When the perceived threat is overwhelming, the freeze response is activated as a last resort. This results in a sudden drop in heart rate and blood pressure, leading to a decrease in cerebral blood flow and fainting. This immobilization and loss of consciousness can be seen as a protective mechanism, allowing the individual to escape psychological distress and emotional pain through a temporary loss of consciousness. This is a very deep-seated subconscious secondary gain, a need to escape emotional pain on a primal level.

Awakening the fainting response is possible. In one study I conducted, my coauthor and I discovered that increasing a sense of safety decreased IBS symptoms and promoted a sense of overall well-being. My research colleague, Dr. Louis Damis, and I termed this the *Central Florida Protocol*; it is a safety-based therapeutic approach to regulate the limbic system.[2] You as a parent can do this at home with the tools I provide in this book and by understanding your role as it relates to catching vibes, secure attachment styles, stress contagion and ANTs.

Creating environments that feel safe and nurturing can help people with anxiety, AI, and GI disorders feel more secure and supported. Words matter, vibes matter, and validation is critical. In a later chapter (Chapter 22), I discuss good (i.e., beneficial) stress. By using the knowledge and tools provided in this book, you can develop strategies to promote emotional and psychological safety, which will enhance vagal tone and empower your child to heal. You can help them create a foundation of resilience and well-being that will serve them throughout their lives.

It's our obligation as parents to help our children find a sense of emotional and psychological sense of safety. When they can sense that they are safe, they can shift into their social engagement system and a return to homeostasis. By acknowledging the states of dissociative, shutdown responses you can encourage them to become more embodied in the present moment. You may even find yourself very shocked that you are in a frozen response. Many mothers I work with are.

Melting the freeze response occurs when we can find awareness of what's happening, often by moving from chest breathing to diaphragmatic/belly breathing. Then, we can move toward thought-restructuring techniques, reframing the stress, and catching the ANTs. Reflective, or active, listening is another way to help your child feel a connection with you, to let them know they are being heard in a safe and validated way, which shifts them into something called social engagement biology, which is another way of saying their nervous system feels safe. In addition, as the child develops the habit of daily prayer and/or meditation, they can use this skill to calm their mind and enhance their sense of safety.

My personal favorite techniques, in addition to emotional and psychological safety, and the ones I use personally, are earthing and grounding. As I mentioned in Chapter 2, science shows that early morning sunlight exposure, without sunglasses, and standing or walking barefoot on the ground 10 to 20 minutes a day will reduce inflammation and enhance your mood.[3] I also highly recommend cold water exposure, like an ice bath or cold shower, for a minimum of 11 minutes per week (see Chapter 12).

These techniques (i.e., sunlight exposure and earthing) are all evidence based, and you will feel amazing once you get in the habit of doing them. If you model them for your children, even if you can't get them to do it, they will be curious. Harping will only make them run away. But you'll be pleasantly surprised, maybe even shocked, at how quickly your mood and your health improve. Because vibes are contagious, your children will want to know what you're doing to improve your mood. Just this morning, my younger daughter sent me a picture of her earthing, with her feet in the grass at 7:00 a.m. I never asked her to take in early morning sunlight exposure or go barefoot outdoors, but she has seen me as I come back from outside belting out a Fleetwood Mac song at top of my lungs and dancing across the house. She also has noticed my refreshed look and energized vibe after a cold ice bath. Now, this daughter takes cold water showers five days a week.

I can't make a 15-year-old do anything, and I certainly won't bully my children into making healthy choices. I want to empower them to make these choices for themselves, so I begin by modeling them. My embarrassing dancing and singing vibes are highly contagious; so is the healing that follows.

The Trauma Effect

Unresolved trauma from the past can also lead a person to develop a freeze anxiety response. For some trauma survivors, no activity successfully channels these sensations, so the nervous system collapses into itself, causing a perpetual shutdown.

Peter Levine, a longtime friend and colleague of polyvagal researcher Stephen Porges, has studied the shutdown response through animal observations and bodywork with clients. In *Waking the Tiger: Healing Trauma*, he explains that emerging from a shutdown requires a shudder, or shake, to discharge suspended fight, flight, or flee energy.[4] In a life-threatening situation, and an opportunity for active survival presents itself, we can wake ourselves up. For example, there are a few things you can do at home to include playful activity: using the swing set at the park; creating art; doing finger painting; making mud pies; perhaps walking, dribbling, or kicking a ball—any activity that allows the child to feel safe while engaging with a trusted human and moving their hands and bodies. This is why I will often take my patients on a walk to the park to use the swing set. Engaging in this type of playfulness pulls them out of the freeze response. These body awareness techniques are so simple, yet powerful, and they can be done at home.

When engaged in body awareness techniques, children move out of their dissociative, shutdown responses and become more present in their bodies. When this happens, they are better able to attend to momentary muscular tension; they can escape the fight, flight, or freeze response. It's difficult to calmly connect to our bodies when we feel utter rage and anger inside.

The freeze response is the ultimate pressure-release valve. And the better we understand it, and provide alternate means of feeling safe, the sooner we can melt the freeze.

Part 4

The Balancing Act

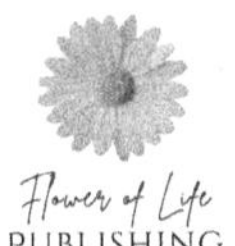

Chapter Fifteen

Family Finances Versus None of Your Business

The hidden cost of stress, something we don't often discuss in public, are money and the impact of financial worries on your sick child's health. By far the most difficult part of my job is when I can't do it. The internal dialogue, the struggle and guilt I feel when I can't help someone because I don't take their insurance and they can't afford the self-pay rate, is heart crushing. The worst part is when they are desperate for relief and I have the answers, but the time, or the money, may not align.

This book and my podcast ("Heal Your Mind, Heal Your Body with Dr. Skyler") were born out of the hope I could reach thousands and provide answers for free, or for the cost of a book. I don't like having a long pro bono wait list because I'll never get to it fast enough to help those people in a timely manner. So, as we get into this chapter, know that, as a single working mom, I understand the pain of the financial burdens having a sick child entails, and I hope to shed light on balancing finances as you embark on the journey of helping your child heal.

Parents who have a child with a severe anxiety, gastrointestinal, or autoimmune condition often face numerous challenges, including the financial burden of medical bills. However, discussing these financial stresses in front of a sick child can have unintended negative consequences, exacerbating a child's stress and illness. So, in this chapter I offer strategies for managing these conversations in a way that supports your child's healing instead.

First, parents must acknowledge the psychological impact of their financial stress, which is felt by their children. Far too often, I hear my patients tell me they feel immense guilt and like a burden for how much their illness costs the family.

In one very extreme case, a 20-year-old male was suicidal and overcome with this guilt. He had to be admitted to a psychiatric hospital several times over a course of a year. The guilt he felt from burdening his parents was too hard for him to bear. He genuinely believed if he were gone from this earth, life for his parents would be all around easier. Guilt, shame, and feeling as though one is a burden occur in 8 out of my 10 of my patients as they begin to realize their role in family finances. Why is this financial stress so prevalent and even life threatening?

In Chapter 4, I discussed your child's sensitivity to parental stress and its impact on their body. Here's a short recap in the context of money.

- *Stress contagion.* Children are highly attuned to their parents' emotions. When parents express stress or anxiety about money, children often absorb these emotions, leading to their own increased stress and worry.

- *Sense of responsibility.* Children, especially those who are already sick, may feel guilty or responsible for their parents' financial worries, believing they are a burden on the family. They have a tendency to be highly empathic and oriented toward people-pleasing.

- *Limbic response.* Financial stress can trigger the fight, flight, or freeze responses in children, leading to heightened anxiety and activation of the dorsal vagal complex (DVC), which is associated with shutdown and immobilization.

- *Declines in health.* Chronic activation of the DVC because of stress can worsen gastrointestinal (GI) symptoms and autoimmune (AI) conditions by impairing digestion, increasing inflammation, and weakening the immune system.

- *Heightened symptoms.* When a child experiences stress from financial worries, their GI and AI disease symptoms can become more pronounced. Stress hormones, such as cortisol, can disrupt the gut–brain axis and immune function, leading to flare-ups.

- *Mental health impact.* The additional stress and guilt caused by finance-related worries can contribute to anxiety, depression, and feelings of helplessness, further compromising the child's ability to cope with their illness. I have treated hundreds of patients with suicidal ideation because they feel like they are a financial burden on their parents.

Why is this so important to your children's health? Back in my generation, we knew our parents struggled with money. They openly talked about it, or they fought about it right in front of us. I recall how awful I felt when I watched my dad come home from work with a handful of bills he had retrieved from the mailbox. I could see the dread across his face. That feeling stayed with me my whole life; I think of him every time I get a bill in the mail. His stress over money had a lifelong impact on me.

We all need money to live. Medical expenses are unreasonably high, and insurance seems to help less and less. But, I ask you, is this financial reality worth exhibiting your stress in front of your children, knowing it makes your child sicker? Or do they need to know what the real world is like so they can be grateful for all your sacrifices? Which one adds more value to their lives over the long term, or can you strike a balance between understanding and protecting them?

Whichever answer best fits for your child's overall long-term health and well-being is the answer. So, what can you do to create a sense of safety despite the costs their illness has placed on your family? Protecting their peace is the bottom line. Here are some ways you can help protect your child's peace:

- *Create a safe environment.* Ensuring that home is a place of emotional safety and stability is crucial. Children need to feel secure and supported, free from the added burden of financial concerns, especially given that they cannot do anything to help, which breeds helplessness.

- *Engage in open communication.* Although it's important to be honest with children, the manner and context in which financial information is shared should be carefully considered to avoid causing undue stress.

- *Have private conversations.* Discuss financial matters privately, away from the child. Ensure that these conversations are held in a calm and solution-focused manner.

- *Use age-appropriate communication.* If financial topics must be discussed with the child, ensure that the information is age appropriate and presented in a way that reassures them of their safety and security.

- *Use positive self-talk.* To combat feelings of guilt and responsibility, teach children to use positive self-talk. Use affirmations like "You are loved," "You are safe," "You are not a burden," and "You are worth it." This is what I told Ella after she had an epic emotional meltdown over her fears about how much money her treatment was costing. I reassured her: "You are my child, and a gift I prayed for. I knew I would have financial responsibilities when I had children. My bills are none of your business, and your health is my priority. We will be mindful of expenses, and it will all work out. It always does." I keep it short now when she starts to get that deer-in-the-headlights, doe-eyed, sad look when I go to pay a balance or co-pay at the doctor's office visits. I tell her to walk away and I say this southern term: "Non-yuun," which is short for "None of your business." Adding humor helps alleviate the reality of it, and I want her focused on her health, not my finances.

Consulting with a financial advisor can help you create a manageable plan for handling medical expenses, thereby reducing the overall stress related to finances. Investigating courses, programs, and resources that provide free mental health services can be helpful. I do have some patients who have traveled outside the country and have reported receiving top-notch medical care with limited out-of-pocket expense.

Overall, financial pressures are a part of life. But they don't have to negatively influence your sick child. Remember, fostering a sense of security, positivity, and resilience in your child is crucial for their healing journey. By managing financial discussions with care and focusing on emotional well-being, you can help your child navigate their health challenges and not feel burdened by adult issues.

Chapter Sixteen

The Glass Child Versus the Sick Child

My sister always had a solid excuse to get out of stuff. I just felt frustrated. She got to sleep late, get out of chores, miss school and I just felt frustrated because I had to pick up more of the slack and do more of the chores and I still had to go to school. I had to help out more. It was a little annoying.

It felt like I was walking on eggshells. Sometimes I'd be careful about what I said and what I did. Everyone was already so stressed, I just didn't wanna add to the burden of it so I just began to stuff my frustration, pain, anger and I became bitter and quiet and more withdrawn. To be very honest, it felt unjust and I was resentful. Then I feel guilty for being mad and then ashamed. She was so sick all the time and with all they (my family) had going on, I felt left out even though I'm perfectly healthy. I felt ignored, like a servant, an errand girl. It's like I'm supposed to be an adult and do adult things to help out.

I'd go out and laugh and have fun, and then I'd feel guilty because my sister can't do all the things I can. It feels like I can't win for being happy and I can't win for carrying the extra physical load and emotional pain.

***

This is a real account from the sibling of one of my patients, and it illustrates *Glass Child Syndrome.*

In families with one child who requires significant medical or behavioral attention, it's common for the siblings to feel overlooked or invisible. The phenomenon of Glass Child Syndrome presents unique challenges and requires mindful intervention to ensure that every child in the family feels seen, heard, and valued. In this chapter, we will explore the impacts of Glass Child Syndrome on family dynamics and provide practical strategies for empowering all children in the household to heal and thrive.

Glass Child Syndrome refers to the experience of children who are often overlooked because another sibling has significant needs due to illness, disability, or behavioral issues. The term "glass" implies transparency: These children feel as though they are seen through rather than truly seen. This dynamic can profoundly affect the emotional and psychological well-being of the Glass Child and the overall family environment. It is natural for parental attention and resources to be unevenly distributed in family that has a sick child. Parents are placed in a position in which they must devote a disproportionate amount of time, energy, and resources to the child with special needs, inadvertently neglecting the Glass Child. This can lead to feelings of abandonment or feeling unloved in the Glass Child. The parents, in turn, experience added emotional strain as they feel torn about where to place their very limited time and energy.

We as parents often experience significant stress due to the demands of caring for a sick child, which can reduce our emotional availability to our other children. Family communication may be disrupted. A lack of open dialogue because of an extreme focus on the sick child might result in limited communication about the Glass Child's feelings and experiences, fostering a sense of isolation. Misunderstandings and conflict may be a common occurrence. Without open communication, misunderstandings and unresolved conflicts can fester, leading to long-term family tension. The following are some of the key characteristics of Glass Child Syndrome:

- *Emotional neglect.* Glass Children may feel emotionally neglected when parental attention and resources are heavily directed toward the sick sibling.

- *Identity struggles.* They may struggle with their sense of identity and self-worth, feeling valued only for their ability to help or remain unobtrusive.

- *Suppressed emotions.* To avoid burdening their parents, Glass Children may learn to suppress their own emotions and needs. This is the most common characteristic I see.

- *Self-worth issues.* The feeling of being continually overlooked can lead to low self-esteem and identity issues.

- *Achievement patterns.* They might either overachieve, to gain attention and approval, or underachieve because of a lack of support.

- *Resentment and jealousy.* The Glass Child might feel jealous or resentful toward the child who is receiving more attention and care, which can strain sibling relationships.

- *Protective behavior.* Conversely, some Glass Children might become overly protective or nurturing toward their sibling with medical needs, taking on a pseudo-parental role.

- *Increased risk.* Glass Children may be at increased risk for anxiety, depression, and other mental health issues because of emotional neglect during formative years.

Growing up as a Glass Child involves a complex mix of emotions that can shape the child's identity and relationships. Life can be an emotional roller coaster for the Glass Child. Their emotions often fluctuate between love, resentment, guilt, shame, and responsibility because parental attention and resources may be unevenly distributed. The emotional strain and the stress of caring for the child's medical needs can diminish parents' emotional availability to their other children. One of the most pervasive feelings a Glass Child experiences is the sense that they are being overlooked. When parents' attention is predominantly focused on a sibling with special medical needs, it's easy to feel invisible, as if their achievements and struggles don't matter. Watching a sibling receive more attention, time, and resources because of their medical needs can breed jealousy and a strong sense of unjustness. It's not that Glass Children resent the siblings, but the uneven distribution of parental attention can be hard to process and even lead to feelings of guilt. They know their sibling's needs are legitimate, yet their longing for equal attention makes them feel a sense of selfishness or ungratefulness.

Alongside resentment, many Glass Children develop strong protective instincts toward their siblings. This can lead them to take on a caregiving role, further blurring the lines between sibling and parent. To avoid adding to their parents' stress, a Glass Child will often suppress their own emotions and needs. This self-silencing can lead to a buildup of unexpressed emotions, which can affect mental health. Without a safe space to express these feelings, they might struggle with emotion regulation and openness in other relationships.

Impact on Sibling Relationships

Siblings play a crucial role in the family, especially when one child has significant medical or behavioral needs. The relationship between a Glass Child and their ill sibling is multifaceted, characterized by deep bonds and underlying tensions. As they bond through shared experiences and grow up together, they develop a unique understanding of each other's challenges. This can create a deep, empathic bond. During collaborative play, the Glass Child often learns to adapt their play and interactions to accommodate their sibling's needs, fostering creativity and patience. Conversely, tensions and conflicts arise. Unspoken resentments and unresolved feelings of jealousy and neglect can lead to unspoken bitterness, creating underlying tension in the relationship. Parents may intervene in an attempt to smooth over conflicts, but this can sometimes unintentionally exacerbate feelings of unfairness and neglect.

Not often thought about is the impact of a sibling's illness on the Glass Child's navigation of their social circles as they explain their siblings' illness to friends and teachers. Social interactions often involve explaining their sibling's condition to friends and peers, which can be a source of both pride and frustration. Carving out their own, individual identity that is separate from their sibling's needs can be challenging for a Glass Child, especially when those needs are often seen in the context of the family situation.

The psychological and emotional effects of being a Glass Child are profound and can influence their development and mental health, particularly as related to their self-worth and identity issues. They may demonstrate validation-seeking behaviors such as becoming overachievers, striving for validation and recognition. Or they may struggle with identity confusion, balancing their own identity with the role they play in their sibling's life. Anxiety and depression may result from suppressed emotions and the constant need to support others while sacrificing their own needs. The pseudo-parental role and the pressure to be perfect can lead to burnout, affecting their academic and social life.

Conversely, Glass Children may experience positive attributes, including learning resilience and enhanced empathy. The experience of being a Glass Child often enhances the child's empathy and understanding of others, making them more compassionate individuals. Problem-solving and conflict resolution skills increase as they adapt to their sibling's needs.

Raising a child with a medical illness, as well as a Glass Child, adds more complexity to an already-full plate for parents. I would be remiss if I did not include some tools to help with the often-neglected and unspoken family dynamics involved in raising a child with health concerns. Healing and growth for a Glass Child require intentional support and strategies to address the emotional and psychological impacts. So, the following are some strategies parents may find helpful:

- *Ensuring balanced attention.* Parents can be mindful and strive to balance their attention, ensuring the Glass Child feels seen and valued. Regular one-on-one time can make a significant difference. Even setting aside 20 minutes a week for uninterrupted one-and-one time will make a huge difference.

- *Offering validation and support.* Validating the Glass Child's feelings and providing emotional support helps them feel understood and less isolated. They may feel immense guilt and resentment all at once, and this is a huge source of shame and pain for them.

- *Providing safe spaces for expression.* Creating safe spaces for them to express their feeling of resentment, unfairness, and guilt without fear of adding stress to the family dynamic is crucial.

- *Encouraging hobbies.* Encouraging them to pursue their interests and hobbies helps them develop a sense of self, and personal achievement is also critical. What do they like to do to bring themselves happiness?

- *Celebrating achievements.* Taking time out to celebrate their milestones and achievements, no matter how small, and reinforcing their values and individuality, will help build their autonomy and distance themselves from their role as a Glass Child.

Raising a Glass Child involves navigating a complex emotional landscape, balancing love and responsibility so they do not feel neglected and build resentment. By understanding and addressing these dynamics, parents and caregivers can create a more balanced and supportive environment. Ensuring that every child feels seen, heard, and valued is essential for their emotional and psychological well-being. Glass Child Syndrome can significantly affect family dynamics, creating blind spots of emotional and psychological challenges for everyone. Being aware of this dynamic is the first step. With this knowledge, parents can pursue balancing attention, open communication, and supportive interventions to foster a healthier, more inclusive environment for all of the family members.

I also recommend professional support. In today's modern society, typically we don't have extended family members living down the road to help raise the kids and listen to their woes. Even if it "takes a village" to raise a child, we simply can't rely on that village to help meet the emotional and psychological needs of our children. That's why I value having an adult role model who provides a judgment-free zone for your child to vent. Mental health issues need not be present—an ounce of prevention, right? We all deserve to feel heard, safe, and understood. It's OK if you don't have the time or bandwidth to meet all of your children's needs at once. That's life; that's parenthood! Instead, think like an emergency room doctor and provide what I call "triage care," tending to the one who has the most urgent needs at the time and then mindfully tending to the others.

Chapter Seventeen

Are You Trauma-Bonded to Your Child?

This chapter is the scariest one for me to put into print. It's the big pink elephant in the room, but it has to be discussed, or else it can have crushing long-lasting effects. I know I've given you a lot to digest. Challenging our thoughts, parenting, and attachment styles can be a very humbling experience.

As if caring for a sick child is not enough, a whole new batch of complex dynamics can occur after your child heals from a chronic illness. The way some parents on occasion feel when all their prayers have been answered may surprise you, or it may even hit home on a deep, hidden, secret level. While raising a sick child, parents can form a *trauma bond*—an emotional connection that develops between two people based on shared traumatic experiences—with the child. This can lead to *enmeshment*, a dynamic in which family members are emotionally reactive to one another and intertwined in an unhealthy way. For example, a child can be emotionally "parentified," which is when the child cares for the parent's emotional needs. For example, a mother might tell her teenage daughter about her issues with her husband, in the hope of feeling connected and not so alone.[1]

Another common experience is when parents feel unneeded and unsure how to transition into a healthy parental role when they are no longer needed as much.

Unfortunately, being trauma-bonded to your child can lead to another phenomenon I have experienced professionally, as have many other therapists: when a parent becomes threatened by the therapist. This is a form of trauma bond that can create a sense of dependency and intense emotional attachment. Trauma bonds often form as a survival mechanism, whereby the individuals involved rely on each other for support and safety during difficult times.

It's humbling, and can be embarrassing, when someone else knows all your flaws and some exaggerated ones based on your child's perspective. We have all, even mental health professionals, yelled or cursed, lost our cool, said something regrettable. It's awkward, but please know, I don't judge the patient's parents. Most therapists don't. We know parents are doing the best they can, and it's not my place to judge anyone, ever. Our job is to provide safety and empower our patients, as best we can, with the knowledge and tools to navigate life. It becomes second nature not to judge.

So, for all the parents who are worried that the therapist is judging you, we don't. We take data set points of information from all the stories to help best treat your child. I must include this chapter because I see this too often in unhealthy attachment styles when the child has healed and the parents do not evolve with the child. If I had a nickel for every time a teen tells me they will be better once they are out of the house, I'd be able to retire now. So, let's go there; let's dive into the elephant of therapy no one talks about: the enmeshment and fear that your child's therapist has some sort of magical hold on your child.

When their child's condition improves, or heals altogether, some parents become unsettled as their new role in the relationship changes and the child no longer requires as much time, attention, or nurturing. But the hiccup comes up when a parental insecurity arises, as the parents come out of the feelings of desperation and are awakened to the realization that someone else knows their parenting flaws. They think, *My child must have told the therapist all these horrible things about me* and *I feel like I am losing control over my child.* Or it may sound like, *My child is more bonded to their therapist than to me.*

These are normal thoughts and to be expected. The challenging part is when the parent has this realization, feels threatened, and abruptly pulls the child out of therapy.

In some cases, the insecure/anxious parenting attachment style loops its way back around after the child has healed and the parents have lost a sense of purpose. The parents are no longer needed as much as they once were. The child's self-efficacy has grown, their anxiety has declined, and boundaries are drawn to protect their peace. Parents fear they have lost connection to their child, or a sense of purpose, and they may feel intimidated and take it out on the child in an inadvertent way, worried the child is more bonded to the therapist.

To ease all the minds out there, they are not more bonded to their therapist. Spending 1 hour a week—4 hours a month, at most—does not erode your years of 24/7 primary caregiving.

We professional therapists know how to monitor what is called *trans-ference*, a phenomenon in which a patient or client seems to direct their feelings or desires related to an important figure in one's life—such as a parent—toward someone who is not that person: the therapist.[2] In short, transference happens when you project feelings about someone else onto your therapist. A classic example of transference is when a client falls in love with their therapist. However, one might also transfer feelings of rage, anger, distrust, or even dependence. Therapists spend years in training learning how to master this phenomenon, and we redirect the bond back to the family if it's safe to do so, or we create space to address transference and work through it. If it's not safe to redirect a bond back to the family, such as in the case of an unhealthy environment, we seek other family support for the child or increase their resilience and coping skills.

Parents take their young adults or late teens out of therapy when they realize they may have revealed family secrets, or the parent feels insecure, or the parent feels they can no longer influence the older child or even young adult in the direction they want them to go. They feel they have lost control over and influence on the child, even a young adult child who is leaving for college. When this occurs, an unfortunate outcome results for the child. For example, they may seek greater independence and move out so they can continue to get even better while exploring their new life. Or they may distance themselves from their parents in other ways and never trust the parent again but rather placate them until they are financially independent. On the other hand, the child may continue to expect the same level of attention, a form of a secondary gain.

There is no doubt that post-healing dynamics lead to a shift in roles. The child gains more independence, and the parent's role as a caregiver diminishes. This transition can be challenging for parents who have dedicated themselves to their child's care. The shift can evoke feelings of loss, uncertainty, and even a sense of purposelessness. The child is in a secure therapeutic bond with the therapist, and this leaves the parent feeling threatened.

Understanding enmeshment is key. As mentioned earlier in this chapter, an enmeshed relationship is one in which boundaries between individuals are blurred, leading to over-involvement in each other's lives. In the context of chronic illness, enmeshment can develop as parents become deeply integrated into their child's care and emotional world. Parents may have difficulty distinguishing their own needs and emotions from those of their child. They might overidentify with their child's experiences and struggle to allow the child independence.

Enmeshment can hinder a child's development of autonomy and self-efficacy. The child may feel overly dependent on their parents and struggle to make decisions independently. Parents may experience heightened anxiety about their child's well-being, even after recovery. This can lead to overprotectiveness and difficulty accepting the child's newfound health and independence. A child who recovers from a chronic illness may wish to explore new activities and assert their independence; however, an enmeshed parent may struggle to let go, constantly checking on the child and expressing concerns, thus stifling the child's growth.

Feeling unneeded is a common parental reaction to a child's recovery. Their identity, which was closely tied to caregiving, is now challenged. Parents may subconsciously harbor feelings of anger or resentment toward their child—or the therapist—for getting better, because it disrupts the established family dynamic and leaves them feeling adrift. The parent may feel threatened, lost, helpless, confused, upset, mad, jealous, resentful, or scared, and then ashamed and guilty for not being thrilled that their child is healed. A different stress rises, and arguments may increase as, subconsciously, the parent tries to re-create the insecure attachment or even the trauma bond they may have shared with the child while they were sick. As humans, we try to re-create the trauma in our life so we can try to resolve it. Our brain tries to close a loop of pain. Re-creating pain and trauma happens in all facets of life.

Breaking the trauma bond can be painful for you as a parent. This is temporary, and nothing to judge yourself for. By bringing awareness to it you can begin to heal in multiple areas of life and create a deeper, healthier bond with your child. I always recommend that caregivers seek support, so they have a safe place to cry and break down, a place to be held emotionally.

Understanding the dynamics of a trauma bond is essential because it has the potential of impacting the well-being of both the child and the parent in several ways. Emotional symptoms include overwhelming attachment. The parent and child may develop an overwhelming attachment to each other: The child feels unable to cope without the parent's presence, and the parent feels indispensable to the child's well-being. Fear and anxiety are present. Both child and parent may experience heightened fear and anxiety about the child's health, leading to a continual state of hypervigilance and stress. The constant emotional strain of maintaining a trauma bond can lead to burnout, depression, and anxiety for both the parent and child—followed by guilt and shame.

The child may feel guilty for being a source of stress and worry for the parent, and the parent may feel shame for their inability to alleviate the child's suffering. The parent also may feel shame and guilt for wanting the trauma bond or deep emotional connection to remain. The parent struggles with how to create an emotional connection with their child outside of the disease. No one needs Mama like a sick kid, and it feels so rewarding when our children need us on such a primal level, like cuddling a sleeping baby.

Behavioral symptoms include overprotectiveness. The parent may limit the child's ability to engage in normal activities out of fear for their health. Conversely, the child may become overly dependent on the parent, struggling to perform tasks or make decisions without the parent's involvement.

Common cognitive symptoms include *catastrophic thinking*, in which one is always anticipating the worst possible outcomes regarding the illness. Distorted perceptions are present as well. The intense focus on illness can distort perceptions of normalcy, and both the parent and child may find it difficult to envision a life beyond the medical condition.

I worked with my daughter Ella to replace our illness bond with a new shared interest. We love to travel, so I used shared lived experiences as a means to reconnect on a new level. But this can also be achieved by going on walks, playing cards or board games, simply doing something interactive. Take a deep interest in your child's newfound interests. You will be very surprised what you learn about your child once they are healed and can speak up for themselves.

There is a consequence for not attempting to create a new neural pathway after the illness. Trauma bonds can limit the child's personal growth and development because the parents' overprotectiveness and dependency hinder their ability to develop autonomy and self-efficacy. The intense focus on managing the illness can lead to social isolation for both parent and child because their world revolves around medical issues. The chronic stress associated with trauma bonds can exacerbate the child's medical condition, leading to flare-ups and worsening symptoms. For the parent, chronic stress can also lead to health problems, such as hypertension, fatigue, and a weakened immune system.

Healing the trauma bonds includes fostering independence and encouraging autonomy. Gradually encourage your child to take on more responsibilities and make decisions related to their care and daily activities. This helps build their confidence and sense of independence. Empower your child by involving them in activities they can complete that can help them feel more in control and less dependent on you as the parent. I have found that grocery shopping is a huge confidence booster, and it is something we all do. Many kids love the empowerment of helping make selections that are based on the criteria set by the parents.

Establish healthy boundaries between you and your child to ensure that you both have space to grow and develop independently. This might involve setting aside time for your self-care and individual activities. Seeking the help of a therapist or counselor can be beneficial in establishing boundaries and addressing the emotional dynamics of the trauma bond.

Encourage open and honest conversations with your child about the challenges and emotions you both are experiencing. This can help reduce misunderstandings and promote mutual support. Validate each other's feelings and experiences without judgment. This can strengthen the emotional bond in a healthy way and reduce the sense of isolation.

Promoting resiliency, as you may recall from Chapter 16, allows normal, unpleasant stress to provide good-stress (called *eustress*) challenges. Take on challenges you both can complete and bond over. Shift the focus from the illness to positive aspects of life. *Celebrate small victories and effort over outcome.*

Navigating trauma bonds in the context of illness requires a delicate balance of empathy, support, and independence. By understanding the nature of these bonds, and implementing strategies to foster healthy relationships, you can break free from the cycle of dependency and emotional strain.

Although the healing of a child is a cause for celebration, it can also present emotional and psychological challenges for you both. Understanding the complexities of enmeshment, recognizing your emotional reactions, and promoting healthy role transitions are crucial steps in fostering a supportive and balanced family environment. It took work to care for the sick child; now it simply takes a new form of awareness to be healthy after they are healed.

Chapter Eighteen

Repurposing the Pain

Pain is an inevitable part of the human experience, but how we interpret and respond to it can profoundly influence our healing journey. Pain can either refine or define us. As a mind–body expert who has healed from an autoimmune (AI) disease by harnessing the power of the mind, I have witnessed firsthand the transformative power of finding meaning in pain. When we resist pain, it becomes suffering. I embrace the importance of finding meaning in suffering, drawing on concepts from faith, spirituality, and psychological practices to offer insights and practical strategies to individuals facing chronic illness and pain. Immense healing over the course of your life awaits as you embrace the concept that pain has purpose. Shedding light on the darkness of pain, giving it meaning, helps your child answer the question "Why me?"

Recall from Chapter 10 Holocaust survivor and psychiatrist Viktor Frankl, who was among the first to study how to find meaning from suffering. He developed logotherapy on the basis of the premise that finding meaning in life, even in the most difficult circumstances, is crucial for psychological health. He argued that humans are primarily driven by a "will to meaning." Finding meaning in suffering can serve as a powerful coping mechanism, helping individuals transcend their pain and find a sense of purpose and hope.[1]

People who find meaning in their suffering often exhibit greater resilience, enabling them to navigate their challenges with strength and optimism. Research has shown that a sense of purpose can improve mental health, boost immune function, and enhance overall well-being, contributing to better health outcomes for those with chronic illnesses.[2]

However, repurposing the pain cannot be forced. It is discovered; it comes from deep within. This *knowingness* is independent of feelings; it's an uncomplicated process that yields a profound sense of certainty. It is a sense of something greater than oneself. So, parents must hold out hope that meaning will come. We like to say, "Someday this will all make sense," when a child is in pain. You can also plant a seed with something like, "When you feel up for it, let's imagine how someday this experience could have greater meaning for you and others."

I am not suggesting that suffering from abuse is warranted. If you are anything like me and the millions out there, we have to acknowledge that "it" happened, and we can't change that. They did what they did, you felt what you felt, and it is what it is. We can only heal, grow, learn, and get back out there to cultivate a love for life again. The same goes for your child. You've gone to great lengths to help your child avoid any pain and suffering, yet it still happened. So, now what?

Start with accepting the fact that your child's medical issues have affected them, you as the parent, and the family dynamics in many ways. This is now a part of your journey and life story. But I don't take this step lightly. Accepting is, by far, the hardest concept to come to terms with during the entire process of raising a child with AI and GI disorders. But we have to remember that if all obstacles were removed from our entire lives, would we have learned the lessons and the wisdom we have now? Memories that lose their emotional charge become wisdom.

Acceptance is a form of surrender, which is, ironically, very empowering. It's not feeling powerless over the outcome, which breeds fear and despair. The pain can serve a purpose as the parent accepts their role as a shepherd guiding their child through the journey—not fixing or trying to control their child's illness.

What do I mean by "surrender?" Buddhists struggle with this concept, as do people of all faiths, as well spiritual believers. So, why am I now asking you, a parent of a child with an anxiety, AI, or gastrointestinal (GI) disorder, to surrender to the process? Because if you've gotten this far into the book, you realize you have no control other than over your own emotions. You have no real sense of power, and that creates more pressure to obtain power and control. But you *can* be helpful. You can still surrender to the process and be helpful by being present and mindful and calmly walking alongside your child, controlling what you can. This may include not arranging for too many doctor appointments in one day, not having the news blaring, not arguing about money in front of them, and regulating your vibes. Control what is in your realm, but if you try to control, or fix, all of it you will only increase your own stress and anxiety, which can bleed onto the child, making matters worse.

Parents can be helpful without being controlling. What does that look like? It looks like this: empowering your child with a belief system that they can trust themselves, that they can heal themselves, that you are there to be a beacon of light so they don't crash on the rocks, that you have the strength and the stamina to quietly use the power of silence to simply listen. When they are sobbing on the bathroom floor, begging for a normal life, you can ask, "What can I do for you at this moment?" This is not the time to talk, or to offer life advice. Just quietly hold the space as they release the stress. The parental instinct is to tell them, "Sshhh, don't cry, it's OK; stop crying." This is code for "Your crying makes me uncomfortable." This creates a belief in your child that they are not safe to feel the moment. The goal is to empower your child to feel and express themselves so you can validate them as a human going through pain.

Here are more empowering statements and questions to provide a sense of safety during the pain and suffering:

- "What can I do to help you feel safe?"
- "I am here; I've got you."
- "We will get through this together as a team."
- "We can figure this out together."
- "You are safe. It's OK that you don't feel OK now."

Feeling safe is all your child has ever wanted since birth. Parents can be the pillars of calm, safe confidence.

Spiritual Perspectives on Suffering

Suffering can also be a powerful way to connect with the Divine, God, or a Higher Power. In moments of pain, a person may find solace and strength in their faith, experiencing a sense of spiritual awakening and connection. Practicing mindfulness, prayer, and meditation can help you become more aware of your child's thoughts and emotions, fostering a deeper understanding of suffering and its potential meaning. When you practice these, you ground yourself while modeling that for your child and your intentions and energy become contagious. One of my proudest moments was walking into my teen's room and seeing her meditating in secret! She wouldn't have ever told me—it's a teen thing, especially when your mom is a therapist. My children don't want me to know they actually listen to me so they can emulate me, but that day my daughter admitted she had been meditating for months.

For your child, keeping a journal in which they reflect on their experiences of pain and suffering can help them identify patterns, insights, and potential sources of meaning in their struggles. However, don't read their journal; it must remain private. One of my other all-time-favorite tools, which I practice nightly, is cultivating gratitude, even in difficult times. This helps me shift my focus from what is lacking to what is present and find meaning and appreciation in their journey. In the 1990s, researchers at the HeartMath Institute identified a physiological state called *heart coherence*, defining it as a type of resonance that occurs when our body's systems, our breathing, heart, and brain rhythms and hormonal responses, are in alignment. This research demonstrated that writing five things you are grateful for each night increases vagal tone and heart coherence.[3]

The concept of heart coherence is rooted in the idea that the heart and brain communicate in a dynamic, ongoing relationship and that the heart's rhythms can directly influence emotion states and overall physiological functioning. Heart coherence is associated with feelings of calm, well-being, and emotional stability. Achieving heart coherence involves consciously focusing on positive emotions, such as appreciation, gratitude, or love, which in turn affects the heart's rhythm and enhances communication between the heart and brain.

When the heart, mind, and emotions are aligned and in sync, this state is characterized by a smooth, balanced heart rate variability pattern and is associated with a sense of well-being and emotional stability. Research shows that heart coherence has a significant impact on reducing anxiety and improving gut health. The connection between the heart and the gut is facilitated by the vagus nerve, which plays a crucial role in regulating both the digestive system and emotional responses.[4]

Experiencing chronic illness has heightened my empathy and compassion for others facing similar challenges. By connecting with and supporting others, I have found a profound sense of meaning and community. In my own journey with an AI disease, I found meaning by seeing my pain as a call to deepen my understanding of the mind–body connection and to help others heal. This shift in perspective transformed my suffering into a source of purpose and fulfillment.

There are several ways you can repurpose pain:

- *Service to others.* When I focused on others, I made a way to get out of my own way. Lying around overthinking my problems created bigger problems. Engaging in acts of kindness in service to others can provide a sense of purpose and fulfillment, reinforcing the meaning found in suffering. In service to others we are forced to see outside of our limited paradigm, our microcosm of misery. Serving others oftentimes feels selfish because when it's done right, it feels good.

- *Spiritual practices.* Faith, hope, and prayer have been studied within the field of *neurotheology,* which explores the relationship between spirituality and the brain, and there is evidence to suggest that these practices can have significant positive effects on health. Hope and faith are powerful psychological tools that can bolster the immune system. Research has shown that people who maintain a sense of hope and purpose have better immune responses.[5] It has also shown that those who engage in regular prayer or have strong spiritual beliefs report lower levels of pain and better pain tolerance.[6] This is thought to be due to the way faith can alter pain perception in the brain, providing a sense of comfort and reducing the emotional impact of pain. The limbic system, including the amygdala and hippocampus, is crucial for emotion processing and memory. The amygdala is involved in the emotional intensity of experiences, and the hippocampus is related to memory formation. These areas are often activated during spiritual experiences, linking emotions with the sense of the Divine or sacred. The most successful cases I have treated, including Ruthie (see Chapter 2) and dozens of others, have achieved healing that is beyond my comprehension as a clinician. The patients in my most successful cases had faith or a belief in the universe, God, or the Divine incorporated into their mind–body practices. Perhaps the main reason I am still healed and thriving is because I have spent my life in service to others as a form of grateful repayment for all my blessings. And for me, it's in service to God.

- *Gratitude journaling.* Expressing gratitude has been shown to activate the parasympathetic nervous system, which is responsible for the body's rest-and-digest functions, improving heart coherence. It is also associated with a reduction in systemic inflammation, including in the GI tract. Listing three things a night that you are grateful for is all it takes to start a real shift. I understand that it sounds simple, but it does work, and that's why it's part of Therapy 101.

Finding meaning in suffering is a powerful and transformative process that can significantly enhance healing and well-being. By drawing on concepts from faith, spirituality, and psychological practices, a person can reframe their pain into purposeful meaning, fostering resilience, growth, and a deeper connection to themselves and others. Embracing the journey of finding meaning in suffering is a vital component of holistic healing and a path to a more fulfilling and balanced life.

Part 5

The 8 Mind-Body Methods to End Anxiety, GI, and AI Conditions

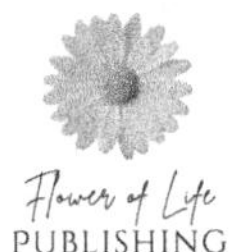

Chapter Nineteen

Safety-Based Protocol Steps 1–4

Start With the Scientific Interplay Between Mind and Body

My Safety-Based Protocol integrates neuroscience and psychology and is the foundation upon which I built my eight mind–body methods to empower your child to heal from troubling anxiety, autoimmune, and gastrointestinal conditions. The first four methods focus on science-backed truths about how the body reacts to anxiety, along with my suggestions for using those truths to our advantage. If you've read all the way through this book, you will notice that the methods discussed in this chapter have been mentioned before. But I wanted to give this summary as a quick tutorial you can refer to often.

By the way, you can access and share my Safety-Based Protocol by visiting https://drskyler.net/8-mind–body-methods.

1—Regulating Emotions Promotes Healing

Emotions are fundamental to the mind–body connection; they serve as the glue that binds our mental and physical experiences. Therefore, emotion regulation is essential to healing because how we feel influences our physiological responses, affects our immune system, and plays a critical role in the development and progression of diseases.[1] Emotions trigger reactions through the autonomic nervous system, which regulates involuntary physiologic processes, including heart rate, blood pressure, respiration, digestion, and arousal.

Psychoneuroimmunology (PNI) is the field that studies how thoughts and emotions influence the immune system. Positive emotions can enhance immune function, and chronic negative emotions can suppress it, making the body more susceptible to illness. Emotions such as joy, love, and gratitude can trigger the release of beneficial neuropeptides and hormones, enhancing cellular function and promoting health. In contrast, emotions such as fear, anger, and sadness can result in the release of stress hormones like cortisol, which can suppress immune function and contribute to inflammation and disease. This means that our emotional experiences can directly alter cellular functions. In short, emotions can either promote health and healing or contribute to the onset of illness and disease.

Dr. Bruce Lipton, a cellular biologist, has explored how emotions and beliefs influence our biology. He emphasizes that our perceptions and thoughts can influence the cellular environment. Lipton's work in epigenetics demonstrates that genes are not the sole determinants of our health; instead, our environment, including our emotional and psychological states, can modify gene expression.[2]

Emotions are more than feelings. Science, along with the field of PNI, has demonstrated why internal or external stress factors, our core beliefs, and automatic negative thoughts (ANTs) all affect immune responses and overall health. Thoughts create emotions, and emotions create thoughts. This bidirectional relationship is influenced by stress. So, the most important mind–body method to heal is to regulate emotions. Of course, this is easier said than done.

Start by understanding the role of emotions; be curious about them, holding no judgment for them. This puts our feelings into perspective. Next, we need to allow ourselves to feel and find a healthy way to express those emotions. Emotions come and go, and expressing them helps flush them out faster. An unexpressed emotion becomes a mood, which can last for days and weeks on end and affect those we love most. So, avoid allowing emotions to build up. Emotions can be buried alive if they remain unexpressed, and they will come out to haunt you at the most inconvenient time. Whether positive or negative, acknowledge them; hold no judgment for them; express them either verbally, if possible, or write them down, even if you throw the paper away—just get them out. We're seeking homeostasis, a balance, by limiting the highs and lows that emotions create. I provided more details in Chapter 4.

2—Turn Your ANTs Into Automatic Loving Thoughts

Building onto the first mind–body method is the second one. Our thoughts have a profound impact on our emotional and physical well-being. A 2005 article from scholars at the National Science Foundation summarized the existing research, which suggests that the average person thinks 12,000–60,000 thoughts per day. This research also suggests that 80% of these thoughts are negative, and 95% are repetitive. That equates to nearly 10,000–48,000 negative thoughts per day! Because our thoughts influence our emotions, we have to learn how to transform ANTs into automatic loving thoughts (ALTs). ANTs are involuntary and often irrational, and they can perpetuate stress and anxiety. They are spontaneous and usually go unnoticed. They often involve distorted thinking patterns such as catastrophizing, overgeneralizing, and negative self-talk. Persistent ANTs can lead to chronic stress, contributing to the onset and exacerbation of gastrointestinal (GI) and autoimmune (AI) conditions. For instance, a child with a chronic illness might constantly think, "I'll never get better," which can heighten anxiety and worsen their symptoms.

Start by catching ANTs before they spread. By observing when an ANT arrives, we can learn to recognize it and do something healthy with it. I suggest transforming ANTs into ALTs. Instead of thinking "I'll never get better," try "I love that my condition is temporary. I will overcome this."

3—Develop Immunity to Stress Contagion

Chronic stress can lead to prolonged activation of the body's survival mechanisms, resulting in hormonal imbalances and inflammation, which are key factors in the development of chronic diseases. Conversely, positive beliefs and emotions can promote a state of relaxation and healing, supporting the body's natural regenerative processes. I've discussed the wide range of internal and external sources of stress and anxiety we face in today's modern society. Plus, studies show stress is contagious, being transmitted through social interactions, especially within families.[3] A child's stress can increase if they sense their parents' anxiety about medical bills or their condition, exacerbating their symptoms. Stress is not only a personal experience but also a social one.

Chronic stress is the enemy of our well-being. We have to learn how to protect our peace so our children can protect theirs as well. I have addressed many ways to approach this core concept in Parts II and III.

4—When Your Mind Is in a Limbic State, Your Body Is in Limbo

Recall that the limbic system, in particular the amygdala, is involved in detecting and responding to threats. It triggers our natural fight, flight, or freeze survival mechanism, which works great when we are temporarily facing danger. But if the limbic system is chronically triggered, remaining in a heightened state of alert, our immune system becomes compromised, which can lead to the development or worsening of diseases due to increased inflammation, digestive disruption, and immune system suppression.[4]

The limbic system also stores emotional memories, such as past traumas. These memories can be triggered by present-day circumstances, which can release the limbic system's fight, flight, or freeze response as if the memory were brought back to life in that moment. For children with chronic illness and past traumatic medical experiences, the limbic system can lead to heightened anxiety and stress in future medical situations.

Knowing about the limbic system is the first step to getting your body out of a state of limbo. But additional steps can be taken to reduce, even eliminate, these chronic stressors. Refer back to Part III for more details.

These first four mind–body methods to empower your child to heal are backed by science as well as my own personal and professional experiences. Regulating our emotions, monitoring and changing our thoughts, and learning to manage stress provide a solid foundation for my Safety-Based Protocol, allowing us to heal from anxiety, GI, and AI disorders. The next four methods focus on the psychology of healing and reframing our behaviors to support healing. When we put this chapter together with the next one, and implement them in our daily lives, we remove insecurity while increasing our ability to heal our body and its correlating stress responses. We soon will be creating immunity to threats to our safety.

Let's get into the psychology of healing now.

Chapter Twenty

Safety-Based Protocol Steps 5–8

LEARN TO LEVERAGE THE PSYCHOLOGY BEHIND HEALING

Understanding the psychological factors that influence the disease process is the basis for the second half of my Safety-Based Protocol. In this chapter, I explore the remaining four methods that embody the mind–body connection and explain the psychological influences on attachment styles, chronic invalidation, secondary gains, and the healing phases. These psychological factors contribute to the development and management of chronic illness, particularly in the context of anxiety, gastrointestinal (GI), and autoimmune (AI) conditions.

5—Attachment Styles That Help or Hurt Healing

Attachment theory, developed by John Bowlby, explains how early relationships with caregivers shape our emotional and social development. These attachment styles influence how we respond to stress and form relationships throughout life. I covered these in more detail in Chapter 5.

- *Anxious attachment (aka the Bulldozer or Helicopter parent).* People with an anxious attachment style have a fear of abandonment and intense emotional responses. This style can lead to heightened stress and anxiety, impacting physical health.

- *Avoidant attachment (aka the Avoidant parent).* This attachment style is characterized by emotional distance and self-reliance. Avoidant individuals may suppress emotions, and they may refuse to let others to express theirs, which can lead to chronic stress and associated health problems.

- *Fearful–avoidant attachment (aka the Disorganized Parent).* This is a mix of two attachment styles and is characterized by a lack of a coherent coping strategy, often because of trauma. This attachment style is associated with higher levels of stress and a greater risk of developing psychosomatic illnesses.

- *Secure attachment (aka the Lighthouse parent).* This attachment style is characterized by trust and a sense of safety. People with secure attachment are generally better at managing stress and have healthier coping mechanisms.

6—Why Chronic Invalidation Prohibits Healing

Chronic invalidation occurs when an individual's feelings, thoughts, or experiences are consistently dismissed or ignored by others. This can happen in family dynamics, social interactions, or medical settings. Chronic invalidation can lead to feelings of worthlessness, depression, and anxiety. It undermines self-esteem and can contribute to the development of mental health disorders. The stress and emotional pain caused by chronic invalidation can manifest in physical symptoms, including GI and AI conditions. Chronic stress from invalidation can disrupt the gut–brain axis and weaken the immune system.

Patients with chronic illnesses often report feeling dismissed or not taken seriously by health care providers, which exacerbates their stress and symptoms. Children who grow up in environments where their feelings and experiences are invalidated may develop chronic health issues because of the prolonged stress and emotional turmoil.

Parents can turn this around by using active listening and validating what they are hearing. This is not the time to fix your child's problem: Just listen, empathize with how they are feeling, and seek to understand what they are going through. See Chapter 5 for more information on this topic.

7—Be Aware of Secondary Gains

Secondary gains are the indirect benefits a person receive from being ill (see Chapter 7 for details). These can include attention, sympathy, financial support, or relief from responsibilities. Think of a secondary gain as a subconscious pressure cooker relief valve. Although the primary gain of being sick might be symptom relief, secondary gains can unconsciously reinforce the illness. The benefits associated with being unwell can create a psychological barrier to recovery. Secondary gains can perpetuate illness by reinforcing the role of sick person. Children may find it difficult to recover if they feel that being well would lead to a loss of support, or to increased responsibilities. Understanding secondary gains while reserving judgment or direct confrontation about them will benefit you and your child in the long run.

A common secondary gain from illness is not attending school or completing homework assignments. Your goal as the parent is to decrease the value of the secondary gain without overt commands or threats; instead, validate and relate without judgment. For example: "I can imagine it may sometimes feel good to miss school. I can understand that. When you're ready, I will be. too."

8—Moving Through the Phases of Healing

When sick with a GI or an AI condition, a person subconsciously goes through phases of healing, and can be in any of these phases at any time. These phases include the Martyr, Victim, Survivor, Thriver, and Warrior, and they were elaborated on in Chapters 9 and 10. Each phase can occur at any time in life, not just during times of trauma or sickness, but your child typically will exhibit signs of being in one phase or the other. The goal is to help them move through each phase until they reach the Warrior phase. During stressful times, a particular phase may become more exaggerated. With the benefit of self-awareness, insight, and the courage to be vulnerable, most of us can identify when we in a particular phase.

The Victim and Martyr phases are most closely associated with the disease progression process with the infiltration of automatic negative thoughts (ANTs); negative core beliefs; and the feeling that one is a captive of one's own mind and body, with no sense of a way out. In these two phases, the person does not take accountability for their role, thoughts, words, or actions in the healing or disease process. What sets a Victim apart from a Martyr and from becoming a Survivor on the way to healing is accountability. When we can hold ourselves accountable for our role in the disease process, we switch from a mindset of being a victim of our reality to being the creator of our lives. You can't force your child out of the Victim or Martyr phases, and please don't call them out; instead, model for them what you would like to see for them. Take gentle accountability for your role in your own ANTs and your own stress contagion, and create moments to build accountability and self-efficacy. Promote the effort of your child's actions, not the result.

Once a child can feel accomplished, they begin to want more. Even grocery shopping builds resilience and self-efficacy. Therein lies the shift—a desire to feel better internally.

Developing awareness of your own ANTs can help your child build awareness of their own. Remember, emotions are contagious; so are healing phases. Birds of a feather flock together; we are who we spend our time with. So, ask yourself, are you a victim of your life, or are you taking accountability, challenging your ANTs, protecting your peace and spreading automatic loving thoughts and peace? Is your attachment style creating a reality for you independent of your role as parent? If you can model the Survivor and Warrior phases, your child can follow you.

Chapter Twenty-One

The Power of Language and Silence

Words Can Sabotage or Empower Your Child to Heal

Words offer significant power and energy that can either benefit your child or be a detriment to helping them heal. Therefore, your language and word choices become essential tools that shape your child's thoughts, emotions, and behaviors. Remember, your child's identity is not their diagnosis or disease. Their physical state is only a small fraction of the human they are growing into. And the words we choose influence who they are becoming.

In Chapter 8, I introduced the influence of neurolinguistic programming, a psychological approach that explores the connection among neurological processes, language, and behavioral patterns. Simply put, the words we choose influence our children's emotions and resulting physiological responses. This chapter delves further into these principles, and the importance of words and linguistics in the disease–wellness process, and offers practical strategies for leveraging language and silence to promote health and healing.

Your words hold more power than you can ever imagine. Ask yourself this: Did your parents' words leave a lasting impression on you? Now, you have the power to modify your language and shift your child's energy and perspectives. Vibes are contagious, and words hold power. Positive language promotes well-being and supports the immune function, whereas negative language can exacerbate stress and illness. Either way, language influences our internal dialogue, or self-talk, which plays a crucial role in shaping our beliefs and behaviors. Positive self-talk can enhance resilience and coping, whereas negative self-talk can undermine confidence and health. That's because linguistics in the mind–body connection shape our perception of reality. The way we describe our experiences influences how we feel about them and react to them. For instance, describing pain in catastrophic terms can intensify the sensation and distress. On the other hand, reframing these descriptions, even being playful, can reduce the sensation. Beyond that, I've observed that patients who use positive, hopeful language about their condition are more likely to engage in healthy behaviors and adhere to treatment plans.

Sometimes, it's the words we don't say that are most helpful. I call this the *Power of Silence*. When a sick child is emoting through their words, it's tempting for parents to chime in with what they assume will be helpful. However, this can have the opposite effect. It's a balancing act, but parents need to learn when to just listen in silence, bearing the pain alongside their child. Silent listening sends the message that you are, in fact, listening and trying to understand what they are feeling and going through. Being heard feels validating. Even if you don't necessarily agree with what they are saying, you can relate to their human condition, understanding that they want a loved one to talk to.

Nine times out of ten, your child just wants to feel understood and know they are not alone. They simply want you to hold a quiet, safe space. If my kids need me to just listen, and get something off their chest, I squirm at times, wanting to say something. But I reply with silence while being attentive with eye contact. Try to avoid saying, "I understand," because in reality you don't. When it's your turn to swap roles from listener to speaker, simply say something like, "I can only imagine how difficult this has all been," or "Thanks for telling me; I'm here for you," "It's important to me that I understand what you are going through; thanks for telling me," or "I'm always here if you ever need me."

To build on the power of silence, I suggest using verbal and nonverbal *mirroring* and *matching* techniques to enhance your communication loop. These involve subtly mimicking body language, tone, and language patterns to create a sense of connection and understanding. These techniques feed a subconscious rapport that can do wonders. For example, if you notice your child physically leaning into the conversation, try leaning in as well.

Serving as a complement to the power of silence is active listening. Active listening allows the person to feel connected, understood and heard. This technique demonstrates that you are fully engaged in the conversation, reflecting their word choices and feelings and validating their experiences. Active listening doesn't mean adding your own thoughts, feelings, or advice; instead, it entails confirming that you hear and understand what is being said. Sometimes, your role as the parent role is to be the listener and to demonstrate your care as an active participant.

Language Includes Modeling

Your child is watching you, and in most cases they admire you. As a result, they will repeat your behaviors and word choices because they want to be just like you—even if only subconsciously. So, parents who model positive language techniques will see their children communicate in similar ways while reminding them of the hope that they can enjoy life beyond their disease or anxiety.

If you model kindness and respect with your words and the way you listen, your child will mirror that back. I am shocked at how many parents disrespect their kids and defend how they speak to them because they are "the parent" and unhappy with their child's behavior when their own sassy, disrespectful tone is mirrored back to them. That baffles me. These children learn to expect the parent to get snappy, and they learn that if they reply in a similar way they will get in trouble. It's akin to when your spouse snaps at you; do you send sunshine and rainbows their way? We can expect the same from our children.

However, if you model emotion regulation and respect even when you are furious, you are demonstrating emotional intelligence, which your child will learn. You can be furious, but you have healthy ways to express it.

Imagine your child being spoken to by their partner the way you are speaking to them: Would you want your child in a relationship like that? Would you be proud they married someone who speaks to them the same way you speak to them when you are angry? If this is a tough question to answer, or it offends you, it may hold some truth. I'm not trying to upset you, but I am trying to shed light on reasons why some children experience anxiety, depression, and health issues. If we want our children to be respectful, we must model respect. The way you talk to them now will influence what they will tolerate in the future. One thing is sure, what we learn as children is what we will tolerate as adults. And what—and how—we communicate is what will be repeated.

Chapter Twenty-Two

The Power of Belief, Finding Flow

When I was healing from multiple sclerosis, I developed a motto. It may sound a little harsh, but it's what helped my mind shift from sick victim to healing survivor. It was, "So what? You are not dying." I would often have severe pain or numbness in my legs and extreme debilitating nausea and vomiting, as well as blinding migraines that lasted for days. Once I was told that I was not dying from the pain (by my neurologist)—that it's just pain—I began to reframe my approach, my belief, my perception of pain, and the stress that accompanied it, and I made this my philosophy. *"So what? Your leg is numb. Now what? You're not dying. Are you going to spend your life complaining, or go live it!?"*

I had what is called "drop foot." I would go to walk, and my foot would not listen to my brain. I used to get so mad at my body for betraying me. I would say horrible, self-deprecating things to myself and hate my body. After I decided to get better, I would say, "Well, you're not dying," and I'd send my foot some love, crack a joke, and ask it to move. Half the time it wouldn't listen, and I'd start a comedic dialogue, "Pleeeease. . . OK; fine. I'll move it for you this one time," and I'd pick my dragging toes off the ground and position my foot where I needed it. I would send it laughter and compassion. This was a huge shift in my healing process. I stopped hating my body and stopped seeing its lack of cooperation as a bad thing. I alleviated the stress of it all. I refused to make the lack of cooperation of my limbs stressful; instead, my internal dialogue switched to, "Let's make this an, 'OK, you are not dying so what can you do that will build your confidence?' situation."

I live in Florida, and a staple of the Floridan diet are what are called Pub-subs, a Publix grocery store sub sandwich. So, I made the Pub-sub a reward for grocery shopping with no one's help, which was a major task when I was sick because of the traffic, the parking, the bright lights, the noise, the people, and the flood of sensory overload. After I fell one time in the grocery store parking lot on my way inside, rather than feeling shame and self-hate and adding more stress, I said, "Well, I'm not dying, and as a reward I'm getting myself a Pub-sub." I picked myself up off the oil-stained asphalt, laughed, cleaned off the oil from my beige linen pants and cheerfully rewarded myself with a glorious foot-long Pub-sub. The sense of accomplishment was huge. I was in my late 20s and still self-conscious about how I looked hobbling around in public. Rather than hiding in shame and embarrassment, I made the stress from the act of grocery shopping a reward. This "good stress" helped build my self confidence and self-efficacy.

Our beliefs about stress play a critical role in determining its impact on our health. The way we perceive stress can influence our physiological and psychological responses, ultimately affecting disease outcomes.

Our beliefs about stress—not the actual disruption of homeostasis, but the belief about stress itself—affect ourselves. That's because our beliefs can alter our body's response. Viewing stress as harmful can exacerbate its negative effects, whereas seeing it as a challenging opportunity can harness its positive potential. Also, beliefs about stress influence our mental state, affecting anxiety, depression, and overall mental health.

Key research findings in the stress mindset theory noted by researcher Alia Crum and her colleagues shows that people who view stress as enhancing their performance and growth (a "stress-is-enhancing" mindset) experience better health outcomes compared with those who see stress as debilitating (a "stress-is-debilitating" mindset). A positive-stress mindset is associated with lower levels of cortisol, reduced inflammation, and better cardiovascular health. Conversely, a negative-stress mindset can lead to heightened stress responses and an increased risk of chronic diseases.[1]

In the intricate interplay between mind and body, stress stands as both a necessary survival mechanism and a potential trigger for disease.[2] This dual nature of stress, known as the *stress paradox*, significantly affects our physical and mental health, particularly in the context of gastrointestinal and autoimmune conditions. Exploring the stress paradox, delving into the mind–body connection and its implications for disease development and management, will help you frame your beliefs about stress.

Cognitive reframing is a technique that characterizes stress as a good challenge rather than a threat. This involves recognizing the potential benefits of stress, such as increased focus and growth opportunities. Practices like mindfulness and meditation can help people accept stress without judgment.

We can also shift our perceptions to improve stress responses. For example, we can learn this phrase: "The glass is not half-empty or half-full; it's just water in a glass." Or, "We are all hanging on by a thread in life." Well, some people are hanging by one hand, beating themselves up with the other; others are clawing their way back to the top in the desperate hope of getting off the treadmill of life; and some are hanging upside down and singing. It's all a matter of perspective, and your perspective can be a choice.

Let's review a simple definition of *stress*, a widely overused term. Stress is a disruption in homeostasis. It can be broken down into three categories: The first, *acute stress*, is a short-term response to an immediate threat, often referred to as the fight, flight, or freeze response. It involves the rapid release of stress hormones, such as cortisol and adrenaline, to prepare the body to respond to danger.

The second category of stress is *chronic stress*, which occurs when stressors persist over a longer period. Unlike acute stress, chronic stress can have detrimental effects on the body, leading to a range of health issues.

But there is a third category of stress, called *eustress*. This was briefly mentioned in Chapter 17. Eustress is based on the Greek word *Eu*, which means "good." Eustress is a kind of stress that encourages us to try a new hobby, learn new skills, and even step outside our comfort zone. It makes us feel good while we work toward our goals, go through significant life changes, or start new chapters in our lives. It's a stress response that benefits us. Imagine feeling capable of handling whatever life throws at you, without having to panic, overreact, or plan your exit strategy. Eustress is the map to finding that *I'll figure it out* pot of gold.

Eustress differs from acute and chronic stress in several ways:

- It only lasts in the short term.

- It energizes and motivates.

- It is perceived as something within our coping ability.

- It feels exciting.

- It increases focus and performance.

Eustress can be triggered by positive forms of social engagement, resourcefulness, and communal support.[3] In addition, the release of the hormone oxytocin during the eustress response can push people to seek or provide aid.[4] Eustress, in its best form, can induce a state of flow. Like eustress, flow is a focused state that often is induced by a healthy dose of challenge.

The healing power of flow is real. *Flow*, a concept popularized by psychologist Mihály Csíkszentmihályi, refers to a mental state in which a person is fully immersed in an activity with a sense of energized focus, full involvement, and enjoyment. Flow can occur while taking on a challenge, "getting on a role" or performing "in the zone." Not unsurprisingly, a state of flow has psychological and physiological benefits and plays a major role in promoting healing and resilience in people with diseases.[5] Ask yourself, "What eustress or flow state does my child accomplish on a weekly basis?" (Video games do not count.)

An understanding of the flow state and eustress will help explain why it's so critically important to your children's mental and physical health. Not all stress is bad, and believing so exponentially creates and fosters disease. Of all the tools, if you have to pick one, pick eustress and finding a state of flow to help your child overcome anxiety and disease.

Flow is characterized by complete absorption in an activity, a merging of action and awareness, a loss of self-consciousness, and a distortion of the perception of time. A person in a state of flow experience high levels of enjoyment and intrinsic motivation. Flow typically occurs when a person engages in activities that have clear goals, provide immediate feedback, and present a balance between challenge (eustress) and skill level.

Flow is often described as an optimal experience. It is associated with increased creativity, productivity, and well-being. Csíkszentmihályi's research indicates that frequent experiences of flow contribute significantly to overall happiness and life satisfaction.

Flow creates healing and wellness by reducing stress and anxiety by shifting one's focus away from worries and negative thoughts (i.e., the belief that all stress is bad). Mental absorption in an engaging activity promotes relaxation and psychological resilience. Flow induces positive emotions and a sense of fulfillment. This emotional uplifting can counteract the negative emotional states often associated with chronic illness and disease. Flow is also associated with the release of neurochemicals such as dopamine, endorphins, and serotonin. These chemicals enhance mood, reduce pain perception, and promote overall well-being. The positive emotions and reduced stress experienced during flow can boost immune function, supporting the body's ability to fight illness and recover from disease.

It doesn't stop there. Flow, and eustress, can act as a natural painkiller by diverting attention away from pain and discomfort. The neurochemical changes that take place during flow can also reduce pain sensitivity. For people with chronic diseases, frequent experiences of flow can improve quality of life by providing meaningful and enjoyable activities that enhance psychological and physical well-being.

I based my decision to allow my daughter Ella to pursue her love of theater over her schoolwork on this science-backed concept. My decision is still paying healthy dividends to this very day. I knew letting Ella participate in theater activities would enhance her social connections, increase her self efficacy, build her resilience to stress, increase her window of tolerance to being active again, and engage her in a state of flow. When she is designing costumes, especially historical period pieces, it is stressful learning what thread and textiles were available in, for example, 1502, but she's in a flow state, focused on the difficult tasks at hand that bring her joy. Up to this point, I had been playing chess, not checkers. I knew the science showed that if I had to pick one thing to help my child get better, it was getting her over the concept that all stress is bad. Reframing stress and entering a state of flow was my goal. I was tackling two major components of disease: disengaging her limbic system while using flow and eustress to reduce her pain.

I will forever hang my hat and double down on this single concept. It was a major catalyst to my child healing and the same tactic I had used to heal myself. I found my flow from free diving and horseback riding. Helping your child find their flow, and reframing stress as not always being bad, are life-changing concepts. If your child has been video game bound or room bound for years, this will be a challenge. I advise parents of disengaged, video game–addicted children to make plans outdoors, to take them on walks, travel if they can. Take away the devices and play board games. Create movement in their lives to start this journey.

Other examples of eustress and flow include engaging in creative pursuits such as painting, writing, or playing music. These activities stimulate the mind and offer emotional expression. Physical activities, such as dancing or yoga can also facilitate flow. Playing a challenging card or board game with family, going on a hike or a walk, and riding a roller coaster are all examples of activities that can facilitate eustress and flow.

There is also a concept called the *effort-driven reward circuit*. This is a science-backed idea that states you can activate larger areas of the cortex by moving your hands—even more so than other parts of the body, such as your legs or back muscles. Driving that effort-driven rewards circuit are physical activities that involve our hands, in particular activities that produce tangible products that we can see, touch, and enjoy. This may include knitting, crocheting, drawing, baking, or tending a garden. Activities like these involve our hands and offer an effort-driven reward. The brain–hand connection applies to "making things."[6] A hands-on investment offers tangible results that carry meaning for the creator, including effectively meeting emotional challenges and thus ameliorating depressive symptoms to some extent.

Exercise also promotes flow and eustress through physical activity while inducing neurochemical changes that support healing. Help your child identify activities that naturally capture their interest and attention. Incorporate a variety of activities to prevent boredom and maintain engagement. Trying new activities can also stimulate flow by presenting fresh challenges. Create an environment that minimizes distractions and interruptions. A quiet, comfortable space can enhance focus and immersion in the activity. Start with activities that match their current skill level, and gradually increase the difficulty. This ensures that the activity remains engaging and prevents frustration or boredom.

I try not to harp on this too much, but mindfulness—being fully present in the moment—is my favorite tool of all time. Incorporate mindfulness practices into every aspect of your life and your child's life as often possible; even eating a piece of chocolate can be done mindfully. Mindfulness is a skill that requires practice. It reduces distractions and promotes immersion. For example, emphasize the enjoyment of an activity itself rather than the outcome.

Mindfulness encourages flow and reduces performance anxiety. Schedule regular time for activities that induce flow. Consistency helps us integrate flow experiences into our routines, supporting ongoing well-being. Balance flow activities with other aspects of self-care, such as rest, nutrition, and social connections. A holistic approach enhances overall health and resilience.

Promoting positive emotions, reframing beliefs about stress, and creating eustress boosts immune function. Flow contributes to both mental and physical health and can be a powerful tool for supporting healing and fostering a fulfilling, balanced life. Embracing the power of flow is an essential component of a holistic approach to health and wellness. If one tool stands out from this entire book, my prayer is that it is reframing stress and creating flow.

Chapter Twenty-Three

Mind–Body Panic and Anxiety Hacks

I have offered a book's worth of methods to empower your child to heal by reframing stress, changing your language, and deactivating their limbic system, but sometimes we all need a go-to, and literal, bag of tricks that triggers our child's parasympathetic (rest-and-digest) nervous system (PNS) in a pinch.

While helping my own daughter heal herself, I learned there are moments when I need to reach into my bag and pull out one of the following hacks to bring her back to the present moment. I called it my Relaxation Kit, and I would try to always include it in her backpack whenever she left home. If your child is sick, largely because of ongoing anxiety, and perhaps suffers from panic attacks, I suggest building your own Relaxation Kit and keeping it handy regardless of the situation you and or your child are going to experience.

Before recommending the potential contents of your Relaxation Kit, I want to clarify the differences between a panic attack and an anxiety attack. Understanding the distinction attacks is crucial for effective treatment and management. Although they share similarities, they differ significantly in terms of onset, symptoms, duration, and underlying causes.

Panic Attack

Panic attacks typically come on abruptly, often without any obvious trigger. They can occur unexpectedly and reach their peak within minutes. Panic attacks are usually brief, lasting between 5 and 20 minutes, although the aftereffects may linger longer. Panic attacks are associated with a significant autonomic nervous system response, involving a surge of adrenaline and activation of the limbic system's fight, flight, or freeze response. Although they can occur without warning, certain situations or environments that previously triggered an attack can increase the likelihood of future episodes. Panic attacks can also occur when the person is relaxed, feeling a sense of safety, or doing an activity they enjoy. This leaves them feeling confused as to why it came on, a panic attack could be due to a wide variety of reasons.

The symptoms of a panic attack are more physical in nature and can be extremely intense, including one or more of the following:

- Rapid heart rate (tachycardia)

- Sweating

- Trembling or shaking

- Shortness of breath

- Chest pain or discomfort

- Nausea or abdominal distress

- Dizziness or lightheadedness

- Feelings of unreality (derealization) or detachment from oneself (depersonalization)

- Fear of losing control or going crazy

- Fear of dying

These symptoms can be so intense that they are often mistaken for a heart attack or other serious medical condition.

Anxiety Attack

Anxiety attacks tend to build up gradually in response to perceived stressors or threats. They often develop over a period of time. Anxiety attacks can last longer than panic attacks do, ranging from minutes to hours, or even days in some cases. Symptoms are more cognitive and emotional, characterized by excessive worry and fear about potential future events or stressors. Anxiety attacks often involve a cycle of negative thoughts and worries that perpetuate the feeling of anxiety. They are often triggered by specific stressors, such as work, school, relationships, or health concerns. Symptoms can be less intense compared to panic attacks and may include one or more of the following:

- Excessive worry or fear

- Restlessness or feeling on edge

- Muscle tension

- Fatigue

- Difficulty concentrating

- Irritability

- Trouble sleeping (insomnia)

PANIC VS. ANXIETY ATTACKS COMPARISON

Feature	Panic	Anxiety
Onset	Sudden and unexpected	Gradual and often in response to stressors
Symptoms	Intense and physical	Milder and more cognitive
Duration	Short (5-20 minutes)	Longer (minutes to hours or days)
Focus	Physical sensations	Worry and fear about the future
Triggers	Often occur without a clear trigger	Linked to specific stressors
Diagnosis	Panic disorder	Generalized anxiety disorder, other anxiety disorders

The following are my recommended mind–body panic and anxiety hacks.

1—Boost your vitamin B and vitamin D levels.

The first hack is to know your vitamins, B and D, Low levels of these vitamins are linked to anxiety and depression.

- Vitamin D is believed to influence the production of neurotransmitters, such as serotonin, which can affect mood regulation. Low levels of serotonin are often associated with mood disorders, including anxiety and depression. Several studies have suggested a link between low levels of vitamin D and an increased risk of poor mood regulation and an increased susceptibility to anxiety and depression.[1]

- Vitamin B helps in the synthesis of neurotransmitters such as serotonin, dopamine, and GABA, which are essential for regulating mood and anxiety. A lack of vitamin B can impair neurotransmitter production, leading to increased anxiety and mood disorders. Low vitamin B also is linked to depression.

2—Breathe deeply when panic or anxiety knocks.

Panic attacks often involve hyperventilation, which can exacerbate symptoms. Deep breathing helps to regulate the breath, calming the nervous system.

- *How to Do It:* Inhale slowly through the nose for a count of four, hold for count of seven, and then exhale slowly through the mouth for a count of eight. Repeat three to four times until you feel calmer. So, inhale for 4, hold for 7, exhale for 8.

- *Put your belly into it. How to do diaphragmatic breathing:*

Breathing deeply from your belly (the diaphragm), rather than taking shallow breaths from the chest, can activate the PNS, reducing stress and anxiety.

- *How to Do It:* Place one hand on your chest and the other on your abdomen. Breathe in deeply through your nose so that your abdomen, not your chest, rises. Exhale slowly through your mouth.

3—Breathe through a straw.

Put a straw into your Relaxation Kit. Here's why: By constraining the airflow, the straw forces you to take slower and more deliberate breaths, which can help calm the body's fight, flight, or freeze response. It really helps if your smaller child picks their straw out. They can choose from colors and patterns; some have even put stickers on theirs and really personalized them. This has the following benefits:

- *Focuses attention.* Concentrating on breathing through the straw can divert your mind from anxious thoughts and sensations, providing a form of mindfulness.

- *Regulates carbon dioxide (CO2) levels.* Slow, controlled breathing can help maintain proper levels of CO_2 in the blood, which can reduce symptoms like dizziness and lightheadedness often associated with hyperventilation.

4—Ground down.

Grounding techniques by engaging your senses help redirect focus from anxious thoughts to the present moment, reducing the intensity of the panic attack.

- *How to Do It:* The 5-4-3-2-1 technique is when you identify five things you can see, four things you can touch, three things you can hear, two things you can smell, and one thing you can taste. Alternatively, you can use the 3 × 3 × 3 method and identify three smells, three sounds, and three body parts. Even trying to wiggle your second toe is a grounding exercise that refocuses the mind.

5—Chill out with ice water exposure.

Exposure to cold can activate the vagus nerve, which plays a crucial role in regulating the PNS and promoting a state of calm. The sudden cold sensation can act as a shock to the system, helping to disrupt the panic attack. This shock can jolt the autonomic nervous system out of the fight, flight, or freeze mode. Cold water can trigger the mammalian dive reflex, a response that slows the heart rate and conserves oxygen. This can promote a calming effect on the body.

- *How to Do It:*

  - *Splash cold water on the face.* Splashing ice-cold water on your face can help reset your nervous system. Focus on your forehead and the area around your eyes, which are particularly sensitive to temperature changes.

  - *Hold an ice pack.* Holding an ice pack or a cold object against your neck or wrists can provide a similar shock effect.

      ◦ *Use an ice bath for your face.* Placing your face in a bowl of ice water can be a quick and effective way to induce a calming response. Focus on long slow exhales after submersion.

6—Sour candy is a handy distraction.

The intense, sharp taste of sour candy can serve as a powerful sensory distraction, shifting your focus away from the panic attack. The sudden burst of flavor can engage the brain's sensory processing centers, thereby interrupting the panic response and helping to restore a sense of control. Sour candy also stimulates saliva production and frequent swallowing, which can help regulate breathing and reduce hyperventilation.

- *How to Do It:*

  ◦ *Sour candy.* Keep sour candies in your Relaxation Kit. When you feel a panic attack coming on, suck on the candy to redirect your focus. Examples include Warheads, Red Hots, and lemon drops.

  ◦ *Chewing gum.* Chewing sour gum can provide a similar sensory distraction and help regulate breathing patterns. Or you can chew mint gum and sip on cold water to create a powerful minty distraction.

  ◦ *Vicks VapoRub.* Rub small amount on your wrist and inhale.

7—Close one eye for panic attacks.

Closing one eye as a method to manage panic attacks is a technique that leverages sensory disruption to interrupt the panic cycle. Our brains normally process visual information from both eyes to create a single, cohesive image. When one eye is closed, this binocular vision is disrupted, which can cause a temporary shift in focus and perspective. The brain's visual cortex is heavily involved in processing stress- and anxiety-related stimuli. By closing one eye, the visual cortex's typical engagement is altered, which can help interrupt anxiety pathways.[2]

Plus, panic attacks often involve sensory overload. By closing one eye you reduce the amount of visual information your brain needs to process, which can help decrease overall sensory input and calm the nervous system. Closing one eye signals the brain to slow down and relax. This action can engage the PNS, which counteracts the fight, flight, or freeze response that is initiated during a panic attack.

- *How to Do It:* As soon as you feel the onset of a panic attack, close one eye. While keeping that one eye closed, take deep, slow breaths to further calm your body and mind. Try to focus on a single object with your open eye; this can help redirect your attention away from the panic-inducing thoughts.

8—Hum a tune.

Humming stimulates the vagus nerve, which activates the PNS. This helps promote a state of calm and relaxation, counteracting the fight, flight, or freeze response to a panic attack. Activation of the vagus nerve can slow down the heart rate and lower blood pressure, helping to alleviate the physical symptoms of anxiety. The act of humming can divert your attention away from anxious thoughts and physical sensations, providing a form of mindfulness that keeps you grounded in the present moment. The sound and vibration of humming provide a sensory focus, which can help disrupt the cycle of escalating anxiety.

9—Tune in to binaural music.

Binaural beats work by entraining your brain waves to a desired frequency. For anxiety, frequencies in the alpha (8–14 Hz) and theta (4–8 Hz) ranges are most beneficial because they are associated with relaxation and calmness. Listening to relaxing binaural beats can help reduce the levels of cortisol, the stress hormone, in your body. Binaural beats can stimulate the production of serotonin and dopamine, neurotransmitters that play a key role in mood regulation. The rhythmic and consistent nature of binaural beats can help induce a meditative state, making it easier to relax and let go of anxious thoughts.

- *Choose the Right Frequency:*

o **Alpha Waves (8–14 Hz)**: These are ideal for relaxation and reducing mild anxiety.

o **Theta Waves (4–8 Hz)**: These are great for deep relaxation, meditation, and reducing more severe anxiety.

- *Anxiety Relief Song*

It is worth noting a song that has gained significant attention for its calming effects. Called, "Weightless," by the British band Marconi Union, the song was created in collaboration with sound therapists. I mentioned it in Chapter 4. It features a combination of carefully arranged harmonies, rhythms, and bass lines designed to slow the listener's heart rate, reduce blood pressure, and lower levels of the stress hormone cortisol.[3] Studies have shown that listening to this song can reduce anxiety by up to 65% percent and reduce physiological resting rates by 35%.[4]

The song's structure is unique because it lacks a repetitive melody, which helps the brain relax. The rhythm starts at 60 beats per minute and gradually slows to around 50 beats per minute. As you listen, your heartbeat naturally aligns with this tempo, promoting a state of deep relaxation.

10—Smell isopropyl alcohol swabs.

The strong smell of alcohol can act as a sensory distraction that might help interrupt the cycle of anxious thoughts and physical symptoms. These are easy to pack in the Relaxation Kit and will help with any nausea. Smelling something pungent can shift your focus from internal anxiety to an external stimulus, helping to ground you in the present moment.

11—Combine methods.

Combine any of these methods to double the distraction. For example, you could use cold exposure with sour (or mint) candy to deliver an immediate, multifaceted approach to halting a panic attack. Or, close one eye as you do deep breathing exercises to enhance the calming effect.

Relaxation Kit

With these hacks, now you can assemble your daily Relaxation Kit. For cold exposure, you can use ice packs or a small frozen bottle of water or a Ziploc baggie filled with ice. Toss in sour candies, gum, and a large straw. Add alcohol swab wipes and a playlist with relaxation music. Keep this kit in your child's backpack and one in the car for easy access. For diaphragmatic or belly breathing, you only need to practice regularly when not experiencing a panic attack to become more comfortable and confident in using them during an actual episode.

Epilogue: Look At You Now!

When parents and their sick child implement my advice, such as the suggestions I have offered in this book, they experience a shift. First, they recognize that hope has set in. Next, they see signs of healing progress and may even feel some kind of relief. This all adds motivation to continue turning this corner, making positive changes that empower their child to heal. The years of pressure, fears, and worries come to a halt while curiosity and adaptation accelerate. Some moms begin to take their own health more seriously after neglecting their own needs as they cared for the family and sick child.

When your child no longer shows any symptoms, a new normal sets in. Parents have learned to empower their child, and their child blooms right in front of their eyes, without debilitating anxiety and gut issues. Families are free to take vacations, host birthday parties, and get involved in school or community events. You and your child may even use their pain for a purpose, possibly becoming an advocate for others or speaking out about their condition publicly. As they get caught up in the activity, in unexpected hours, the obvious will dawn on them: Their child is better, now a Survivor or Warrior, and all they endured is now a memory.

That's possible for you and your child.

***

Now is the time to encourage your child to truly live their best life. You can join them! It's a great time to bond over a bigger purpose than ourselves. Remember, the power of belief, words, transforming automatic negative thoughts into automatic loving thoughts, encouraging self-efficacy, autonomy, eustress, flow—all of these have transformed your child's past, and now their future. I hope and pray you embrace the tools and strategies shared in this book and trust in your child's innate ability to heal. Together, you can navigate the challenges of anxiety, autoimmune, and gastrointestinal disorders, emerging stronger, more resilient, and more deeply connected. Your unwavering support and belief in your child's potential are the most powerful gifts you can offer on this journey of healing and empowerment.

You have become the compassionate, quiet beacon of strength that delivers safety to your child in an unsafe world. You have empowered your child to heal.

Acknowledgements

The following pioneers in my industry have had a profound impact on my work. I simply would not have become who I am today if it weren't for them.

Drawing on the wisdom of groundbreaking research, spiritual insights, and practical techniques, I aim to inspire and empower parents to support their children in harnessing their innate healing potential. The mind–body connection is a powerful ally that began with neuroscientist Candace Pert, who discovered that emotions are not just abstract feelings but are deeply intertwined with our biology. Molecules of emotion, such as neuropeptides, play a crucial role in the communication between the brain and the body, influencing health and disease.

By understanding that emotions directly affect physical health, we parents can encourage our children to express and process their feelings in healthy ways, fostering both emotional and physical well-being.

The book *The Biology of Belief* is based on Bruce Lipton's insights. Lipton is a cellular biologist, and his work emphasizes that our beliefs can influence our biological functioning. The environment of our thoughts and beliefs can affect gene expression and overall health. We parents can help our children develop empowering beliefs about stress about their ability to heal. By fostering a positive, supportive, validating environment, parents can influence their child's biology in a way that promotes healing.

Dr. Joe Dispenza's research highlights the power of the placebo effect, demonstrating that our thoughts and expectations can trigger real physiological changes. Believing in the possibility of healing can activate the body's natural healing processes. By encouraging our children to believe in their own healing potential, trust themselves, and build flow and self-efficacy, we as parents can harness the placebo effect. This involves cultivating hope, optimism, and a belief in the body's ability to recover.

Utilizing the healing power of connection and safety, polyvagal theory, developed by Dr. Stephen Porges, explains how the autonomic nervous system regulates feelings of safety and stress. The vagus nerve plays a crucial role in calming the body and promoting healing. We can create a sense of safety for our children through a healthy attachment style, validation, supporting autonomy, and providing supportive relationships and environments. Activities that promote relaxation and connection, such as deep breathing, gentle touch, and mindful presence, can activate the vagus nerve and enhance healing.

I also acknowledge David Jahr, my developmental editor and right hand who guided me every step of the way to become a better writer and communicator. His words, prayers, and Psalm readings gave me strength when I was on my knees, overwhelmed. David was more than an editor for me; he was a kind friend and beacon of light during the darkest, hardest hours of my life during the year it took to write this book. David, from meeting you on my birthday to seeing you on my book-launch day on my next birthday, this book kept me going through my grief. "Thank you" isn't really sufficient, but thank you for helping me make a childhood dream happen.

I want to thank my two very supportive, kind daughters for allowing me to share their stories and carrying the weight of extra chores, making dinner, while I worked very long hours. You both took on roles and extra chores to help make our team Piglets 3 thrive. Thank you, my Loves.

Mom, thank you. I asked something BIG of you: to reveal some family skeletons from my childhood perspective, and with true unconditional mother's love you said, "Honey, write *YOUR* story! Tell the world the story *as you saw it*, and if it serves God and helps one person, that is all that is important in this life."

Last, to the broken Unicorn that led me to my own truth, time, and energy because you said I wasn't worth yours. Your words reminded me of MY power, so with deep gratitude, appreciation, and love, I thank you. The renewed drive to serve God became my life's mission after knowing you, and with that, my second book, *Rewiring Your Heart*, which I am writing now, was born.

About the Author

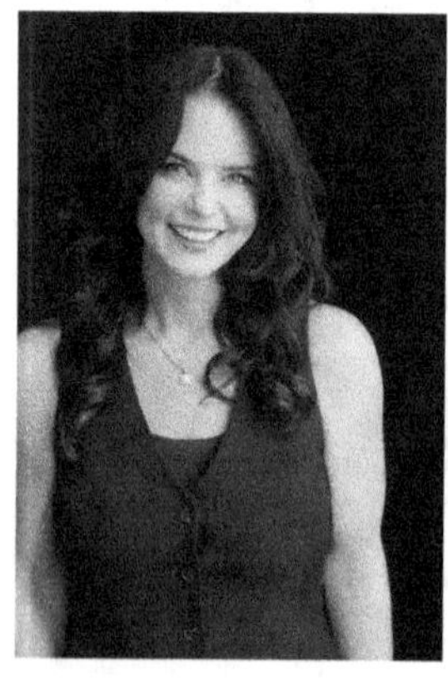

Skyler Hamilton, PhD, specializes in helping people tap into the power of the mind to successfully treat inflammatory diseases, autoimmune and gut–brain disorders, among other complex cases. A mind–body psychotherapist, author, peer-reviewed published researcher, and lecturer, she is an expert on the somatic effects of stress, trauma, and anxiety. A product of her methods, Dr. Hamilton once suffered from multiple sclerosis (MS) and was bound to a wheelchair. With her MS in remission, she now spends her life empowering others to heal themselves with or without medications.

Dr. Hamilton's research on treatment of gut–brain axis disorders with the use of clinical hypnosis has been cited in numerous peer reviewed journals. She lectures on the mind–body connection and its impact on various medical disorders, such as dysautonomia, irritable bowel syndrome, ulcerative colitis, cyclical vomiting syndrome, thyroid diseases, lupus, Lyme disease, mast cell activation syndrome, and juvenile arthritis, among others.

Dr. Hamilton is based in the Orlando, Florida, area, where she lives with her daughters, Ella (17) and Lily (15). In her free time, she enjoys spending time with her family, traveling, and practicing natural horsemanship. She also practices somatic yoga, ice water exposure therapy, scuba, horse riding and deep-water free diving.

Learn more at drskyler.net.

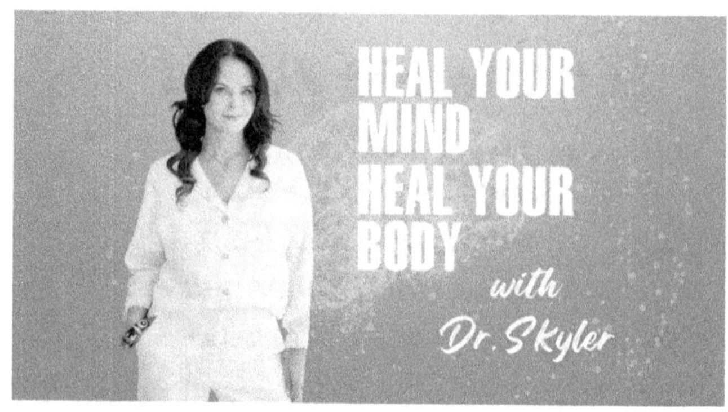

Tune Into Dr. Skyler's Top-Ranked Podcast on your favorite platform, including:

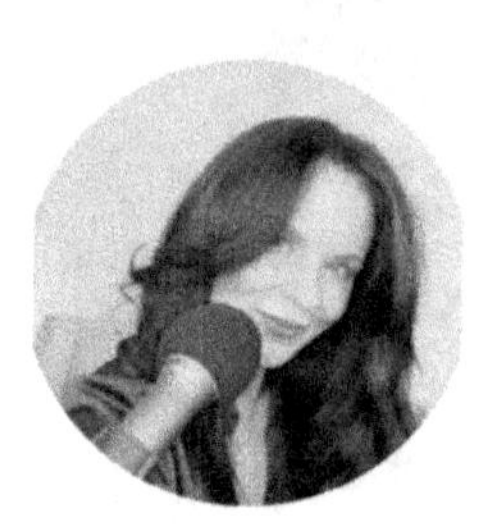

Listen Notes
YouTube: My Gut Response
Apple
Pandora
iHeart
Spotify
Red Circle

Find your favorite episode at:
https://www.drskyler.net/podcast

Want Dr. Skyler as a guest on your show, at your workshop or conference?
https://www.drskyler.net/contact

Endnotes

Foreword

1. Bookwalter, D. B., Roenfeldt, K. A., LeardMann, C. A., Kong, S. Y., Riddle, M. S., & Rull, R. P. (2020). Posttraumatic stress disorder and risk of selected autoimmune diseases among US military personnel. *BMC Psychiatry*, *20*(1), 23. https://doi.org/10.1186/s12888-020-2432-9

2. Hsu, T.-W., Bai, Y.-M., Tsai, S.-J., Chen, T.-J., Chen, M.-H., & Liang, C.-S. (2023). Risk of autoimmune diseases after post-traumatic stress disorder: A nationwide cohort study. *European Archives of Psychiatry and Clinical Neuroscience*. https://doi.org/10.1007/s00406-023-01639-1

3. O'Donovan, A., Cohen, B. E., Seal, K. H., Bertenthal, D., Margaretten, M., Nishimi, K., & Neylan, T. C. (2015). Elevated Risk for Autoimmune Disorders in Iraq and Afghanistan Veterans with Posttraumatic Stress Disorder. *Biological Psychiatry*, *77*(4), 365–374. https://doi.org/10.101 6/j.biopsych.2014.06.015

4. Roberts, A. L., Malspeis, S., Kubzansky, L. D., Feldman, C. H., Chang, S .-C., Koenen, K. C., & Costenbader, K. H. (2017). Association of Trauma and Posttraumatic Stress Disorder with Incident Systemic Lupus Erythematosus in a Longitudinal Cohort of Women. *Arthritis & Rheumatology*, *69*(11), 2162–2169. https://doi.org/10.1002/art.40222

5. Song, H., Fang, F., Tomasson, G., Arnberg, F. K., Mataix-Cols, D., Fernández de la Cruz, L., Almqvist, C., Fall, K., & Valdimarsdóttir, U. A. (2018). Association of Stress-Related Disorders with Subsequent Autoimmune Disease. *JAMA*, *319*(23), 2388–2400. https://doi.org/10.10 01/jama.2018.7028

6. Stojanovich, L., & Marisavljevich, D. (2008). Stress as a trigger of autoimmune disease. *Autoimmunity Reviews, 7*(3), 209–213. https://doi.org/10.1016/j.autrev.2007.11.007

7. Waller, E., Scheidt, C. E., Endorf, K., Hartmann, A., & Zimmermann, P. (2016). Unresolved trauma in fibromyalgia: A cross-sectional study. *Journal of Health Psychology, 21*(11), 2457-2465.

8. Porges, S. W. (2024). Polyvagal Perspectives: Interventions, Practices, and Strategies. First Edition. New York: W. W. Norton & Company.

Why My Child!?!

1. Louis F. Damis and M. Skyler Hamilton. "Impact of Hypnotic Safety on Disorders of Gut–Brain Interaction: A Pilot Study." The *American Journal of Clinical Hypnosis* 63 no. 2 (2020): 150–168. https://doi.org/10.1080/00029157.2020.1794434

2. Stephen W. Porges, "Neuroception: A Subconscious System for Detecting Threats and Safety," *Zero to Three* 24, no. 5 (2024): 19–24.

3. Antonio Berumen, Adam L. Edwinson, and Madhusudan Grover. "Post-Infection Irritable Bowel Syndrome." *Gastroenterology Clinics of North America* 50, no. 2 (2021):445–461. https://doi.org/10.1016/j.gtc.2021.02.007

4. Jeremy Appleton. "The Gut–Brain Axis: Influence of Microbiota on Mood and Mental Health." *Integrative Medicine* 17, no. 4 (2018): 28–32.

5. Rachel Yehuda, "How Parents' Trauma Leaves Biological Traces in Children," *Scientific American*, July 1, 2022. Accessed August 28, 2024. https://www.scientificamerican.com/article/how-parents-rsquo-trauma-leaves-biological-traces-in-children

The Miracle Patient

1. Cristina Stasi, Massimo Bellini, Dario Gambaccini, et al. "Neuroendocrine Dysregulation in Irritable Bowel Syndrome Patients: A Pilot Study." *Journal of Neurogastroenterology and Motility* 23, no. 3 (2017): 428–434. https://doi.org/10.5056/jnm16155

2. Yimin Han, Boya Wang, Han Gao, et al. "Vagus Nerve and Underlying Impact on the Gut Microbiota–Brain Axis in Behavior and Neurodegenerative Diseases." *Journal of Inflammation Research* 15 (2022): 6213–6230. https://doi.org/10.2147/JIR.S384949

The Hardest Part

1. Stefan Schulreich, Anita Tusche, Phillip Kanske, et al. "Altruism Under Stress: Cortisol Negatively Predicts Charitable Giving and Neural Value Representations Depending on Mentalizing Capacity." *Journal of Neuroscience* 42 no. 16 (2022): 3445–3460. https://doi.org/10.1523/JNEUROSCI.1870-21.2022

2. Economic & Social Research Council, "Mum's the Word When It Comes to Children's Happiness," *ScienceDaily*, April 10, 2011, https://www.sciencedaily.com/releases/2011/04/110403090320.htm

3. Stephanie J. Dimitroff, Omid Kardan, Elizabeth A. Necka, et al. "Physiological Dynamics of Stress Contagion." *Scientific Reports* 7 no. 1 (2017): 6168. https:// doi.org/10.1038/s41598-017-05811-1

4. Jamie Schneider, Stress is Contagious — How to Know If You're Catching it, From a Neuroscientist, *MBGHealth*, October 3, 2024. Accessed October 4, 2024. https://www.mindbodygreen.com/articles/is-stress-contagious-50922a#:~:text=According%20to%20Swart%2C%20the%20answer,explains%20on%20the%20mindbodygreen%20podcast.

5. J. A. C. J. Bastiaansen, M. Thioux, and C. Keysers. "Evidence for Mirror Systems in Emotions." *Philosophical Transactions of the Royal Society of London Series B: Biological Sciences* 364, no. 1528 (2009): 2391–2404. https://doi.org/10.1098/rstb.2010.0410

6. Howard S. Friedman and Ronald E. Riggio. "Effect of Individual Differences in Nonverbal Expressiveness on Transmission of Emotion." *Journal of Nonverbal Behavior* 6, no. 2 (1981): 96–104. https://doi.org/10.1007/BF00987285

7. Shawn Achor, Michelle Gielan, Make Yourself Immune to Secondhand Stress, *Harvard Business Review*, September 2, 2015. https://hbr.org/2015/09/make-yourself-immune-to-secondhand-stress. Accessed October 3, 2024.

8. Achor and Gielan, "Make Yourself Immune."

9. Heidi Hanna, *Stressaholic: 5 Steps to Transform Your Relationship With Stress* (New York: John Wiley & Sons, 2014).

10. Achor and Gielan, "Make Yourself Immune."

11. Elissa S. Epel, Elizabeth H. Blackburn, Jue Lin, et al. "Accelerated Telomere Shortening in Response to Life Stress." *Proceedings of the National Academy of Sciences* 101 no. 49 (2004): 17312–17315. https://doi.org/10.1073/pnas.0407162101

12. Achor and Gielan, "Make Yourself Immune."

13. Tori DeAngelis, "Better Relationships With Patients Lead to Better Outcomes," *Monitor on Psychology*, November 1, 2019. Accessed October 3, 2024. https://www.apa.org/monitor/2019/11/ce-corner-relationships

14. Marconi Union, "Weightless," 2011, https://www.youtube.com/watch?v=UfcAVejslrU&ab_channel=JustMusicTV

15. Daniel Shepherd, Michael Hautus, Edmund Giang, et al., "'The most relaxing song in the world'? A comparative study," *Psychology of Music* 51, no. 1 (2023): 3–15. https://doi.org/10.1177/03057356221081169

16. Myriam Verena Thoma, Ricarda Mewes, and Urs M. Nater, "Preliminary Evidence: The Stress-Reducing Effect of Listening to Water Sounds Depends on Somatic Complaints: A Randomized Trial." *Medicine* 97, no. 8 (2018): e9851. https://doi.org/10.1097/MD.0000000000009851

17. Didrik Espeland, Louis de Weerd L, and James B. Mercer, "Health Effects of Voluntary Exposure to Cold Water—A Continuing Subject of Debate," *International Journal of Circumpolar Health* 81 no. 1 (2022): 2111789. https://doi.org/10.1080/22423982.2022.2111789

18. Mihály Csíkszentmihályi, *Flow: The Psychology of Optimal Experience* (New York: Harper Perennial), 2008.

19. Hannah Peach, Jane F. Gaultney, and David D. Gray. "Sleep Hygiene and Sleep Quality as Predictors of Positive and Negative Dimensions of Mental Health in College Students." *Cogent Psychology* 3, no. 1 (2016): Article 1168768. https://doi.org/10.1080/23311908.2016.1168768

What Kind of Parent Are You?

1. Saul McLeod, "Attachment Theory in Psychology," *Simply Psychology*, January 17, 2024. Accessed October 3, 2024. https://www.simplypsychology.org/attachment.html

2. Lisa M. Diamond, Christopher P. Fagundes, and Molly R. Butterworth. "Attachment Style, Vagal Tone, and Empathy During Mother–Adolescent Interactions." *Journal of Research on Adolescence* 22 no. 1 (2012): 165–184. https://doi.org/10.1111/j.1532-7795.2011.00762.x

3. Kylie Agllias. "Missing Family: The Adult Child's Experience of Parental Estrangement." *Journal of Social Work Practice* 32 no. 1 (2018): 59–72. https://doi.org/10.1080/02650533.2017.1326471

196

4. Taishi Kawamoto, Keiichi Onoda, Ken'ichiro Nakashima, et al. "Is Dorsal Anterior Cingulate Cortex Activation in Response to Social Exclusion Due to Expectancy Violation? An fMRI Study." *Frontiers in Evolutionary Neuroscience* 4 (2012): Article 11. https://doi.org/10.3389/fnevo.2012.00011

5. K. A. Davies, G. J. Macfarlane, J. McBeth, R. Morriss, et al. "Insecure Attachment Style Is Associated With Chronic Widespread Pain." *Pain* 143, no. 3 (2009): 200–205. https://doi.org/10.1016/j.pain.2009.02.013

6. Mario Mikulincer and Philip R. Shaver. "An Attachment Perspective on Psychopathology." *World Psychiatry* 11 no. 1 (2012):11–15. https://doi.org/10.1016/j.wpsyc.2012.01.003

Back In "My Generation"

1. Yu Kong. "Are Emotions Contagious? A Conceptual Review of Studies in Language Education." *Frontiers in Psychology* 13 (2022): Article 1048105. https://doi.org/10.3389/fpsyg.2022.1048105

2. Julie R. Ancis. "The Age of Cyberpsychology: An Overview." *Technology, Mind, and Behavior* 1 no. 1 (2020): 1–15. https://doi.org/10.1037/tmb0000009

3. Ancis, "The Age of Cyberpsychology."

Top 10 Things Kids Wish You Knew

1. R. Davidhizar. "The Pursuit of Illness for Secondary Gain." *The Health Care Supervisor* 13 no. 1 (1994): 10–15.

2. Saul McLeod, "Maslow's Hierarchy of Needs," *Simply Psychology,* January 24, 2024. Accessed September 25, 2024. https://www.simplypsychology.org/maslow.html

The Top 5 Things to Never Say to Your Child With an AI or GI Condition

1. "Neuro-Linguistic Programming Therapy," *Psychology Today*, December 5, 2022. Accessed October 3, 2024. https://www.psychologytoday.com/us/therapy-types/neuro-linguistic-programming-therapy

Your Child's Healing Phase(s), Part 1

1. Kevin J. Connors. "Dissociative and Complex Trauma Disorders in Health and Mental Health Contexts: Or Why Is the Elephant Not in the Room?" *Journal of Trauma & Dissociation* 19 no. 1 (2017): 1–8. https://doi.org/10.1080/15299732.2018.1379855

Your Child's Healing Phase(s), Part 2

1. Anthony R. Artino Jr. "Academic Self-Efficacy: From Educational Theory to Instructional Practice." *Perspectives on Medical Education* 1 no. 2 (2012) :76–85. https://doi.org/10.1007/s40037-012-0012-5

2. Nicole Celestine, "4 Ways to Improve and Increase Self-Efficacy" April 9, 2019. Accessed April 16, 2024. https://positivepsychology.com/3-ways-build-self-efficacy/

3. Deb Dana, *The Polyvagal Theory in Therapy: Engaging the Rhythm of Regulation* (New York: W. W. Norton, 2018).

4. "What Is Logotherapy?", The Victor E. Frankl Institute of America, n.d. Accessed April 17, 2024. https://viktorfranklamerica.com/what-is-logotherapy/

The Privilege of Victimhood

1. Birgitta Dresp-Langley, "Children's Health in the Digital Age." *International Journal of Environmental Research and Public Health* 17 no. 9 (2020): Article 3240. https://doi.org/10.3390/ijerph17093240

Deactivating the Limbic System

1. "Gastroesophageal reflux disease (GERD)," Mayo Clinic, accessed September 3, 2024. https://www.mayoclinic.org/diseases-conditions/gerd/symptoms-causes/syc-20361940

2. Gajanon S. Gaude. "Pulmonary Manifestations of Gastroesophageal Reflux Disease." *Annals of Thoracic Medicine* 4 no. 3 (2009):115–123. https://doi.org/10.4103/1817-1737.53347

3. Ikuo Homma and Yuri Masaoka "Breathing Rhythms and Emotions." *Experimental Physiology* 93 no. 9 (2008): 1011-1021. https://doi.org/10.1113/expphysiol.2008.042424

4. Detlef H. Heck, Samuel S. McAfee, Yu Liu, et al. "Breathing as a Fundamental Rhythm of Brain Function." *Frontiers in Neural Circuits* 10 (2017): 115. https://doi.org/10.3389/fncir.2016.00115

5. Tammana Begum, "How Listening to Birdsong Can Transform Our Mental Health," Natural History Museum, October 8, 2020. Accessed September 3, 2024. https://www.nhm.ac.uk/discover/how-listening-to-bird-song-can-transform-our-mental-health.html

6. Carmelita Swiner, "What Are Binaural Beats?", WebMD, April 30, 2023. Accessed October 3, 2024. https://www.webmd.com/balance/what-are-binaural-beats

Landing the Flight Safely

1. Brianna Chu, Komal Marwaha K, Terrence Sanvictores, et al. *Physiology, Stress Reaction* (Treasure Island, FL: StatPearls Publishing). https://www.ncbi.nlm.nih.gov/books/NBK541120/

2. Tone Tangen Haug, Arnstein Mykletun, Alv A. Dahl. "The Prevalence of Nausea in the Community: Psychological, Social and Somatic Factors." *General Hospital Psychiatry* 24 no. 2 (2002): 81–86. https://doi.org/10.1016/s0163-8343(01)00184-0

Melting the Freeze Response

1. Stephen W. Porges, "Neuroception: A Subconscious System for Detecting Threats and Safety," *Zero to Three* 24, no. 5 (2024): 19–24.

2. Louis F. Damis and M. Skyler Hamilton. "Impact of Hypnotic Safety on Disorders of Gut–Brain Interaction: A Pilot Study." The *American Journal of Clinical Hypnosis* 63 no. 2 (2020): 150–168. https://doi.org/10.1080/00029157.2020.1794434

3. M. Nathaniel Mead. "Benefits of Sunlight: A Bright Spot for Human Health." *Environmental Health Perspectives* 116 no. 4 (2008): A160–A167. https://doi.org/10.1289/ehp.116-a160.

4. Peter A. Levine, *Waking the Tiger: Healing Trauma* (Berkeley, CA: North Atlantic Books, 1997).

Are You Trauma-Bonded to Your Child?

1. Sharon Martin, "The Enmeshed Family System: What It Is and How to Break Free," Psych Central, July 26, 2023. Accessed September 2, 2024. https://psychcentral.com/blog/imperfect/2019/05/the-enmeshed-family-system-what-it-is-and-how-to-break-free

2. "Transference," *Psychology Today*, n.d. Accessed September 2, 2024. https://www.psychologytoday.com/us/basics/transference

Repurposing the Pain

1. "What Is Logotherapy?" The Victor E. Frankl Institute of America, n.d. Accessed April 17, 2024. https://viktorfranklamerica.com/what-is-logotherapy/

2. "The Power of Positive Thinking," *John Hopkins Medicine*, n.d. Accessed October 3, 2024. https://www.hopkinsmedicine.org/health/wellness-and-prevention/the-power-of-positive-thinking

3. "What Is Heart Coherence?", HeartMath, September 13, 2022. Accessed September 2, 2024. https://www.heartmath.com/blog/health-and-wellness/what-is-heart-coherence/

4. Rollin McCraty and Maria A. Zayas. "Cardiac Coherence, Self-Regulation, Autonomic Stability, and Psychosocial Well-Being." *Frontiers in Psychology* 5(2014): 1090. https://10.3389/fpsyg.2014.01090

5. Harold G. Koenig, "Religion, Spirituality, and Health: The Research and Clinical Implications," *ISRN Psychiatry* 16 (2012): 278730. https://doi.org/10.5402/2012/278730

6. Alexandra Ferreira-Valente, Margarida Jarego, Inês Queiroz-Garcia, et al., "Prayer as a Pain Intervention: Protocol of a Systematic Review of Randomised Controlled Trials," *BMJ Open* 11, no. 7 (2021): e047580. https://doi.org/10.1136/bmjopen-2020-047580

Safety-Based Protocol Steps 1–4

1. Fulvio D'Acquisto. "Affective Immunology: Where Emotions and the Immune Response Converge." *Dialogues in Clinical Neuroscience* 19 no. 1 (2017): 9–19. https://doi.org/10.31887/DCNS.2017.19.1/fdacquisto

2. Bruce H. Lipton, *The Biology of Belief: Unleashing the Power of Consciousness, Matter, and Miracles.* (Carlsbad, CA: Hay House Publishing, 2008).

3. Ezra Golberstein, Janis L. Whitlock, and Marilyn F. Downs, "Social Contagion of Mental Health: Evidence From College Roommates," *Health Economics* 22, no. 8 (2013): 965–986. https://doi.org/10.1002/hec.2873

4. Brianna Chu, Komal Marwaha, Terrence Sanvictores, et al. *Physiology, Stress Reaction* (Treasure Island, FL: StatPearls Publishing, 2024). https://www.ncbi.nlm.nih.gov/books/NBK541120/

The Power of Belief, Finding Flow

1. Alia J. Crum, Peter Salovey, and Shawn Achor. "Rethinking Stress: The Role of Mindsets in Determining the Stress Response." *Journal of Personality and Social Psychology* 104, No. 4 (2013): 716–733. https://doi.org/10.1037/a0031201

2. Dominik Langgartner, Christopher A. Lowry, and Stefan O. Reber. "Old Friends, Immunoregulation, and Stress Resilience." *Pflugers Archiv: European Journal of Physiology* 471 no. 2 (2019): 237–269. https://doi.org /10.1007/s00424-018-2228-7

3. Peter Suedfeld. "Reactions to Societal Trauma: Distress and/or Eustress." *Political Psychology 18 no.* 4 (1997): 849–861. https://doi.org/10.1111/ 0162-895X.00082

4. Catherine Moore, "What Is Eustress? A Look at the Psychology and Benefits," PositivePsychology.com, January 15, 2019. Accessed September 3, 2024. https://positivepsychology.com/what-is-eustress/

5. Mihály Csíkszentmihályi, *Flow: The Psychology of Optimal Experience* (New York: Harper Perennial, 2008).

6. Cathy Malchiodi, "Drawing on the Effort-Driven Rewards Circuit," *Psychology Today*, August 4, 2008. Accessed September 2, 2024. https://www.psychologytoday.com/us/blog/arts-and-health/200 808/drawing-on-the-effort-driven-rewards-circuit

Mind–Body Panic and Anxiety Hacks

1. Sarah Moore, "The Connection Between Vitamin D and Mental Health," *News Medical Life Sciences*, June 20, 2024. Accessed October 3, 2024. https://www.news-medical.net/health/The-Connection-Betw een-Vitamin-D-and-Mental-Health.aspx

2. Elizabeth A. Phelps and Joseph E. LeDoux. "Contributions of the Amygdala to Emotion Processing: From Animal Models to Human Behavior." *Neuron* 48, no. 2 (2005): 175–187. https://doi.org/10.1016/j.neuron.2 005.09.025

3. Marconi Union, "Weightless," 2011, https://www.youtube.com/watch? v=UfcAVejslrU&ab_channel=JustMusicTV

4. Marconi Union, "Weightless," 2011.

9 798218 529918